# EMOTIONAL DEVELOPMENT IN YOUNG CHILDREN

# The Guilford Series on Social and Emotional Development

CLAIRE B. KOPP AND STEVEN R. ASHER, *Editors*

Children and Marital Conflict:
The Impact of Family Dispute and Resolution
*E. Mark Cummings and Patrick Davies*

Emotional Development in Young Children
*Susanne A. Denham*

# Emotional Development in Young Children

## Susanne A. Denham

*Foreword* by Judy Dunn

THE GUILFORD PRESS
New York    London

*To Nannie, Cal, and Sarah*

*—My motivators*

© 1998 The Guilford Press
A Division of Guilford Publications, Inc.
72 Spring Street, New York, NY 10012
http://www.guilford.com

Printed in the United States of America

This book is printed on acid-free paper.

Last digit is print number:   9   8   7   6   5   4   3   2

**Library of Congress Cataloging-in-Publication Data**

Denham, Susanne A.
     Emotional development in young children / Susanne A. Denham :
foreword by Judy Dunn.
          p.      cm.–(The Guilford series on social and emotional
development)
     Includes bibliographical references and index.
     ISBN 1-57230-352-2 (hardcover : alk. paper).–1-57230-360-3
(pbk. : alk. paper)
     1. Emotions in children. I. Title. II. Series.
BF723.E6D36  1998
155.4′124–DC21                                                  98-24230
                                                                CIP

# Foreword

*T*his is an exciting time to take a close look at the emotions of very young children. Over the last 15 years, what we know of children's expression of feelings, the place of emotions in their development, and especially their understanding of emotions has increased dramatically. We have learned much about how children's experiences at home are linked to their understanding and expression of emotion; we understand, too, much more about how children's relationships with their peers outside the family are linked to their emotional expressiveness, their ability to "regulate" the extremes of their anger or distress, and their grasp of other children's feelings and why they behave the way they do. Much of the key research that has helped to clarify the nature and development of children's emotional understanding and expression has been conducted by separate groups of researchers—experts in rather different fields of psychology, including cognitive development, social relationships, brain-and-behavior links, and the study of serious developmental problems such as autism. Susanne Denham has successfully brought together the core findings and lessons from these various research fields, in a book that is both scholarly and readable, and that includes case vignettes from the real world of children.

She is just the person to clarify the developmental story of children's emotions in the very early toddler and preschool years. I first came across her work in the mid-1980s. Wandering through the hundreds of poster displays in a huge conference held by the American Psychological Association, I happened upon an intriguing poster that described her innovative piece of research on the emotional understanding of two-year-olds. These were children who were much younger than the subjects usually studied by psychologists: the "terrible twos" are clearly not as easy to study as the amenable five- or six-year-olds who were at the time the typical subjects of research of emotions of young children. Yet as I knew from my observational studies of children at home, children of only two years old do react to and manipulate the feelings of their siblings and parents; they know how to tease, comfort, and annoy. It appeared likely that such two-year-olds were certainly more sophisticated in their emotional understanding than their "performance" in conventional standardized assessments would suggest. Denham was among the first to show what these very young children understood; she developed a series of stories played out with puppets that captured these children's interests, and used this strategy to begin the program of studies into individual differences in children's emotion understanding described in this book. Her techniques played a key role in my own longitudinal studies, enabling me to bring together information on children's emotion understanding in standard settings and in their real-life interactions with family and friends. Denham's puppets have now played out their stories not only in the United States but also in London and Cambridge in England, in comfortable middle-class homes, and in tough, inner-city ghettos—and we have learned a great deal from them.

Three characteristics of this book stand out as especially useful. First, the thorough and systematic survey of research on children's understanding of emotions—much of it from Denham's own research team—is full of fascinating findings, such as the evidence on children's understanding of ways to change emotions, and the developmental changes in their grasp of ambivalent or mixed emotions. Her focus on individual differences is particularly welcome and important. Second Denham is sensitive to the *complexities* of the developmental patterns she describes—the puzzles, the inconsistencies, and the questions raised as well as the findings that support her own model. And the questions raised are certainly intriguing. We might ask: What, for example, are we to make of the evidence—often inconsistent—on gender differences in emotional development? or Why should mothers' intimacy and openness of the expression of physical affection be *negatively* related to preschoolers' understanding of emotions?

Third, Denham's model of parental influence on children's emotional development is clearly set out, and the research that supports it is impressive. The lessons for intervention studies will be of interest to anyone concerned with the care of young children. We still have to worry, however, about drawing conclusions about the direction of causal influence, and the processes that underlie the connections between the behavior and emotions of parents and their children remain unclear. (It is possible, for instance, that genetics plays a part in contributing to the links between the emotional characteristics of parents and children, yet this is rarely discussed in models of socialization.) The difficulty of coming to conclusions about the causal influence of parents on emotion understanding was illustrated for me by our findings from a study of families over the period when a second child was born. We found that in families in which mothers *talked* to their toddler firstborn children about the new baby as someone with feelings, needs, and wants, over time both the children (firstborn and baby sibling) behaved in more friendly ways to each other than the siblings in families in which the parents did not talk to their firstborn about the feelings and desires of the baby. This finding led us to a program of research on the significance of children's participation in discourse about feelings. The general pattern of links between early parent–child conversations about feelings and the children's later understanding of emotion and positive relations with other children was replicated in a range of different studies in very different communities. Yet coming to conclusions about whether there were really *causal* connections between parent–child conversations about emotion and children's later developmental outcome remains problematic. It could be that the children in these families where such conversations took place were especially interested in feelings, or particularly friendly with their siblings, and that their mothers were really *responding* to their children's characteristics, rather than causing the developments in the children.

Emotions are at the center of children's relationships, well-being, sense of self, and moral sensitivity and are centrally linked to their increasing understanding of the world in which they grow up. Yet we have only recently begun to pay serious attention to the significance of children's emotions and to the individual differences in emotional expressiveness and understanding that are so striking among young children. This book is especially welcome for its theme, the thorough review of research that it provides, and the many questions that it raises. The place of emotions in the lives of toddlers and preschoolers, not to mention parents, surely deserves our serious attention, and we should be grateful to Susanne Denham for showing us so clearly what we do know and what we yet need to know.

JUDY DUNN, PhD
Institute of Psychiatry, London

# Contents

# 🎭 Chapter 1

# Introduction

*Four-year-olds Joey and Mike are pretending to be pirates. They have rubber swords, cocked hats, "gold" coins, and even a stuffed parrot. They are having a lot of fun. Joey finds the buried treasure–hurray! But then things get complicated, changing fast and furiously, as interaction often does. Mike suddenly decides to be the Queen's Navy, and Joey has to "sword-fight" him. Then Jimmy, who has been nearby, tries to join in. No way! Joey wants Jimmy to leave. At almost the same minute, Mike steps on a Lego and starts to cry. And Rodney, the class bully, approaches, laughing at Joey and Mike for making believe and at Mike for crying. Joey deals with all of them: He comforts Mike appropriately, manages to tell Jimmy to stay out of the game without alienating him, and does his best to ignore Rodney's teasing. When their teacher calls them to have a snack, everybody is satisfied with the morning.*

This is much more than a simple playtime; a lot of emotional transactions are occurring. Joey's clear, convincing, appropriate expressions of emotions aid him in getting what he wants socially:

- When Joey finds the buried treasure, his face shows absolute joy.
- When challenged by Mike as the Queen's Navy, he roars with rage and acts very brave.
- He displays just the right intensity of anger to tell Jimmy to "keep out." Not too strongly, though–Joey doesn't want Jimmy to shout back, "I'm not your friend!"

1

Joey's understanding of emotions also allows him to respond quickly but accurately—to regulate his own emotions and respond to those of others—during rapidly shifting, highly charged play experiences:

- Joey responds to Mike's crying by first quietly giving his friend a chance to pull himself together, and then comforting him. Misinterpreting Mike's grimace as anger could have led Joey to act angry himself, hurting his friend's feelings and endangering their relationship.
- When Rodney comes over, Joey appears noncommittal, masking his anger and fear.

So, within a 5-minute play period, several different elements of emotional competences are called for if the social interaction is to proceed successfully. Taken together, the expression, understanding, and regulation of emotions are vital for determining how Joey gets along with others, how he understands himself, and whether he feels good in his world, within himself, and with other people.

Joey is one "emotionally smart" little guy. Emotional competence like his has only recently received heightened public attention; Daniel Goleman's 1995 book, *Emotional Intelligence,* was even featured on *The Oprah Winfrey Show.* Goleman (1995) alerts us not only to the dire consequences when emotional competence is lacking, but also to the rewards of being emotionally competent—in self-control, zest, sympathy, perseverance, and social acuity. He argues that "emotional literacy" is as vital as any type of learning, and I strongly agree. These abilities continue to develop throughout the lifespan, but preschool-age children are surprisingly adept at several components of emotional competence, including but not limited to the following (from Gordon, 1989, and Saarni, 1990):

### EXPRESSION

- Using gestures to express nonverbal emotional messages about a social situation or relationship (e.g., giving a hug).
- Demonstrating empathic involvement in others' emotions (e.g., kissing a baby sister when she falls down and bangs her knee).
- Displaying complex social and self-conscious emotions, such as guilt, pride, shame, and contempt, in appropriate contexts.
- Realizing that one may feel a certain way "on the inside," but show a different demeanor "on the outside"—in particular, that overt expression of socially disapproved feelings may be con-

trolled, while more socially appropriate emotions should be expressed (e.g., being afraid of an adult visitor, but showing no emotion or even a slight smile).

### UNDERSTANDING

- Discerning one's own emotional states (e.g., realizing that one feels more sad than angry when getting "time out" from one's preschool teacher).
- Discerning others' emotional states (e.g., knowing that Daddy's smile as he comes into the house means his workday was satisfactory, and he probably won't yell tonight).
- Using the vocabulary of emotion (e.g., reminiscing about the family's sadness when a pet died).

### REGULATION

- Coping with aversive or distressing emotions, or the situations that elicit them (e.g., using Mother's assistance instead of immediately resorting to aggression when a younger sibling grabs all the toys, even though one is very upset).
- Coping with pleasurable emotions or the situations that elicit them (e.g., taking a deep breath and downplaying one's laughter even though one is almost uncontrollably gleeful while playing "chase" on the playground).
- Strategically "up-regulating" the experience and expression of emotions at appropriate times (e.g., grimacing in anger to make a bully retreat; singing out loud to share one's enjoyment with a very best friend).

Certainly all these component skills of emotional competence, when functioning optimally, work together in an integrated way. They are intricately interdependent; a preschool girl who is angry and sullen day after day, for instance, is unlikely to learn much about her playmates' feelings. So, although I subsequently describe the expression, understanding, and regulation of emotions separately, it is my hope that the complex interrelations of these components of emotional competence will become obvious. A 5-year-old boy who has successful strategies for regulating anger during a conflict probably recognizes and understands both his own emotions and his friend's, and he probably experiences guilt over causing distress in a friend. The emotion regulation that facilitates this social interaction is built upon a foundation of other aspects of emotional competence.

This integration of emotional expressiveness and understanding within young children's social milieu is inescapable. First, the development of emotion regulation is necessary because of preschoolers' increasingly complex emotionality and the demands of their social world. Their emotional experience becomes more and more complicated as they begin to feel blends of emotions and finely nuanced emotions (e.g., guilt or shame). With so much going on emotionally, some organized emotional gatekeeper—emotion regulation—must be cultivated. Preschoolers' attention is becoming more and more riveted on success with friends, too, and this developmental focus also demands emotion regulation. A crybaby does not fare well on the playground, and a grouch is not welcome during make-believe.

Second, emotion regulation is possible because of young children's increased comprehension of emotionality.

> *Five-year-old Jack can "read" the emotions of his friends. He smiles easily at his friend Allen to cheer him up after a teacher's reprimand, and sneers at the outcast whose sickly smile indicates a bid for play. But Jack can also understand his own emotional signals, and fine-tunes them so he can continue to be the undisputed leader of his group. When he feels a little jittery during small-group time, he tries to still his tapping feet and dancing pencil, because other people (including the teacher) don't like him to behave this way. Besides, he really can do his alphabet work—there's no need to be tense!*

Developmentalists are trying to operationalize these fascinating aspects of emotion regulation—to investigate its emotional, cognitive, and behavioral components.

## THE NATURE OF EMOTION

But wait: What *are* emotions, anyway? Before we delve further into toddlers' and preschoolers' emotional competence, it is important to agree on the nature of emotional experience. The need to define as common a human phenomenon as emotion may seem a bit strange, but the scientific study of emotion has a disjointed history. In initial studies of adult emotion, psychologists carefully pondered their own internal processes. After repeated self-observations, they described their conscious experiences of emotion. So, early in the history of psychology, subjective qualities such as feelings were respectable topics for study.

However, it was admittedly difficult to observe internal states objectively. With behaviorism gaining ascendance in psychology, introspection was no longer considered an acceptable means of study. Only behaviors were investigated, nothing intrapsychic. Phenomena requiring any inferences—such as motivation, thoughts, and feelings—were rejected as unobservable, reducible to overt behavior, and unworthy of scientific scrutiny. Unsurprisingly, due to these converging circumstances, emotions were largely ignored for several decades. They were relegated to the status of afterthoughts—nuisances to be examined when they got in the way of "harder" behavioral science.

Then, with a swing of the scientific pendulum, unobservable psychological internal states were not only deemed acceptable, but seen as central to an understanding of human functioning. Still, however, emotions were overlooked: This revolution in psychology was strictly cognitive, so emotions took a back seat to cognition. In their zeal, cognitive psychologists at first considered emotions mere by-products of cognitive appraisal, and thus not worthy of study in their own right.

More recent innovations in thinking have revised these unbalanced views. Current research suggests (1) that emotion and cognition often work together in the creation of emotional experience—although at times one or the other "takes the lead," neither takes precedence over the other (Lewis & Michalson, 1983); and (2) that emotions are regulators of behavior within oneself (intrapersonal) and in interactions with others (interpersonal).

## What Is Emotional Experience?: Emotion and Cognition Together

There is little disagreement that emotional experience originates with autonomic nervous system arousal, but what happens next is the subject of much debate (see Fischer, Shaver, & Carnochan, 1989; Izard, 1993a; Lazarus, 1991; Stein, Trabasso, & Liwag, 1993). Currently the major disagreement centers on whether cognition determines emotion or not. New research on the brain described by Goleman (1995) and others places many of these arguments in perspective: Sometimes emotion *precedes* cognition, and sometimes it is *preceded by* cognition. These two important systems work in concert, in adults as well as in children. My view of how emotional experiences occur can be seen in Figure 1.1.

First, there is arousal. The autonomic nervous system is aroused by notable change in the person's world. This change can be caused by an environmental event, by the actions of the individual, by the actions of others, or even by memories. Sometimes this arousal is limited to lower, more primitive brain systems. When the "bottom drops out" on a roller-coaster ride, this is certainly a sudden and intense

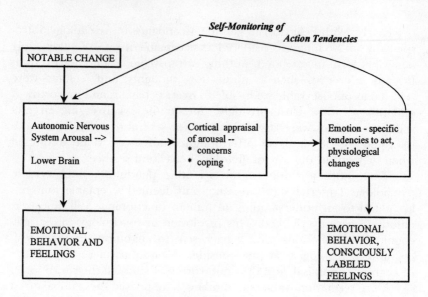

**FIGURE 1.1.** Emotional experience.

environmental change for a 5-year-old girl. And when a 4-year-old boy's mother blocks access to the cookies on the table, her actions are definitely noteworthy. In both instances emotions ensue quickly and automatically, along with their attendant behaviors: The 5-year-old hides her eyes and screams; the 4-year-old glares at his mother and stomps his foot. This process of emotional experience is portrayed in the leftmost column of Figure 1.1.

Individuals experience these lower-level emotions across the lifespan, but after infancy higher brain functioning becomes increasingly important to the nature of emotional experience. From toddlerhood onward, motivation and cognition often work together strongly to influence emotional experience, because individuals create an increasingly complicated network of desired outcomes, or goals. Hence, the need for cortical brain involvement in much of emotional experience is clear: Notable changes and attendant arousal give children important information about their ongoing goals and their ability to cope with events, but this information needs to be *understood*, not just reacted to. A child (or an adult, for that matter) needs to *represent* the notable change, the new thing that has happened. Interpretations of the emotion-eliciting circumstance are necessary. How does the event affect ongoing goals, if at all? Can the child deal with these consequences? These cognitive aspects of an emotional experience are portrayed in the middle column of Figure 1.1.

*As 2-year-old Jessica is playing on the floor, she suddenly sees a large toy action figure, black and rather menacing–certainly unique in her experience–moving into the room on its own. This is a new thing! (Arousal takes place here.) This object must have some sort of effect on her world. But what? (What does this arousal mean? Interpretation is required.) She continues to watch Darth Vader as he comes closer. Slowly she understands that this guy is totally unpredictable. He may interfere with her goal of staying safe. Darth Vader is scary!*

Cognition plays an important role in the emotion Jessica finally experiences. Before any specific emotional reaction is felt by her, or discerned by others, she must attend to the notable event, comprehend it, and interpret it. These interpretations and construals of events' relations to ongoing goals lead not only to felt emotions, but also to actions associated with each specific emotion and to physiological changes in arousal, as portrayed in the rightmost column of Figure 1.1.

In the version of Jessica's experience given above, she feels afraid as a result of her interpretation of Darth Vader's approach (felt emotion). She turns and runs toward her mother, screaming, "I scared" (goal-directed, emotion-related action; labeled feelings). If she finds her mom, her physiological arousal lessens. But if she realizes she is alone, she feels increased arousal instead. So the results of Jessica's emotion-related actions also influence her arousal, and may feed back into new construals and changing emotional experience. As the child matures, self-monitoring of these emotion-related actions and of concomitant changes in arousal comes into play. This pathway is portrayed at the top of Figure 1.1.

Sometimes the precise experience of emotional arousal depends on *which* of several goals the child focuses on. For instance, Jessica may have two goals–having fun and remaining safe. The approach of Darth Vader may affect either goal or both of them. If she cannot remain safe, Jessica will feel afraid. If Darth Vader looks like an interesting toy, she may feel happiness.

In these ways, the argument of whether emotion is predominant over cognition in emotional experiences, or vice versa, can be resolved on the basis of the newest brain research (LeDoux, 1993). Some emotional experiences do not involve cognition; they are mostly automatic. But because the cortical path to emotion predominates after about the middle of the first year, this intimate union of cognition and emotion is usually what is referred to when emotions are discussed (Izard, 1991; Stein et al., 1993). The conceptions of emotion put forward in Figure 1.1 thus will inform the rest of this volume.

## Emotions as Regulators of the Behavior of Self and Others

Another important new way of looking at emotions, which is not at all antithetical with the above-described focus on a child's goals, accents the *functions* of various emotions (Izard, 1993b). What do emotions *do* for children and the people with whom they interact? They provide both the children and others with information (see Campos & Barrett, 1984). This information is important to a child, because it can shape his or her behaviors after or during the experience of emotion. Emotions also affect the behaviors of others, because their expression can help in the effort to describe and predict the child's behavior. So emotions are important both interpersonally and intrapersonally.

Most importantly, the experience and expression of emotion signal that the goal-directed behavior of the child or other people needs to be modified or continued. An example is fear.

*If Marco experiences fear when Billy arrives at day care, the experience of fear gives him important signals that affect his subsequent behavior. He avoids Billy, seeks the lap of a caregiver, and remains vigilant during his day. Marco's expression of fear gives important signals to other people that affect their subsequent behavior, too. His caregivers are watchful because they wish to know what is bothering him, and Billy also studies him, ready to take advantage by grabbing a toy.*

Joey's "pirate" play, described earlier, is likewise replete with evidence of emotions' links to his ongoing goals. When he is happy about finding the buried treasure, his experience of happiness makes him want to continue this enjoyable activity. At the same time, his expression of joy tells his friend Mike that it is an opportune time to join Joey in flinging "gold doubloons" in the air.

First, then, the experience and expression of emotion can affect the behavior of the feeling person. And, second, emotions are important because they provide social information to other people.

*Eighteen-month-old Amy expresses anger when she wants to maintain the freedom to run around the room, but this freedom is curtailed by her parents. She does not want to get into her highchair; in fact, her goal is to continue to dash from the window to the door and back again. Because she experiences this anger, she is likely to engage in specific behaviors, such as kicking and yelling, in service of the goal of freedom. As for her parents, Amy's kicking and yelling lets them know that she does not like the restriction of the highchair. The parents react to this signal with distractions such as singing, or, in contrast, yelling at her to sit still. Peers and siblings, too, benefit from witnessing Amy's expression of emotion.*

*When Amy's 3-year-old brother witnesses her social signal of anger, he may know from experience that his most profitable response is to retreat.*

There is no doubt that the emotional expressiveness of others is a powerful interpersonal regulator, and that this social side of emotion is important. Some prominent researchers and theorists go even further to assert that this interpersonal function of emotion is central to the very nature of emotional expression and experience (Gergen, 1985; Russell, 1989). Saarni (1987) states that "emotion's meaningfulness is grounded in human relationships . . . transactions among people [are] the primary focus for feelings to be experienced, observed or inferred, talked about, and elaborated into expectancies for guiding one through future interpersonal interactions" (p. 536). Thus, even very young children learn the "feeling rules" of their community from their own experiences and the socialization of adults—what to feel in differing situations, how to interpret and manage these feelings, and how to react to the feelings of others (Hochschild, 1979).

## DEVELOPMENTAL CHANGE IN TODDLERS' AND PRESCHOOLERS' EMOTIONAL COMPETENCE

The age period from 2 to 5 years is a time of change for children and caregivers alike. Progress in all areas of children's development—talking, thinking, running and jumping, and playing together—seems to occur daily. Adults are often delighted with these new abilities, especially children's growing deftness in interacting with both grownups and peers.

As amply described above, these new proficiencies are not limited to isolated language, cognitive, social, and motor skills. Children from 2 to 5 years of age are more emotionally sophisticated than we ever previously imagined. The many changes in emotional competence during this age period have prompted developmental psychologists to try to describe them more fully, and to search for the contributions of socialization and maturation to such change. This new focus is particularly auspicious, because it signifies an increasing ability to describe specific children, and to predict their behavior, in terms of physical, social, cognitive, *and* emotional attributes.

Accounts of any child's behavior are arid and incomplete unless they include information on emotions. The important question "What changes over time?" cannot be answered fully without details about children's emotional lives. Children obviously reason in a more abstract way, and become more motorically adept as development proceeds.

But knowing about developmental change in emotional competence—that 2-year-olds' negativity generally wanes considerably, or that kindergartners are at the threshold of understanding finer complexities of emotional experience—is invaluable to filling out a picture of whole children.

There are important implications of these age-related changes. Different levels of emotional competence from children who differ in age should be expected, often because of advances in language, perspective taking, and other social-cognitive abilities. In a group of young children, older preschoolers' expression and understanding of emotions differ from toddlers', and even from younger preschoolers'. A 4-year-old at the playground with her mother, upon seeing another child crying, is no longer so likely to freeze, or even to cry herself, as she was at 18 months. Instead, she is likely to look concerned and ask, "Why is he crying?"

The upper limit of this age range—around the transition to kindergarten—is often a time when children experience growth in their understanding of the causes and consequences of emotions, and in the complexity of their emotions. During a busy day in kindergarten, two boys may discuss who is sitting at, and who is missing from, their snack table. They may commiserate over their shared emotions: "John is here. That's the happy thing." "But Darryl is not, and that's the sad thing. We need to find him on the playground." Another 5-year-old may assert, "Only our moms know what we really feel on the inside." Still another may smile wanly when offered an unfamiliar food by her favorite aunt, instead of refusing it with an ill-tempered retort.

## INDIVIDUAL DIFFERENCES IN EMOTIONAL COMPETENCE

Normative change in emotional competence, although important, does not tell the whole story. Caregivers often unwittingly focus on critical individual differences in children's emotional competence: "She gets upset so easily. I wish I could help her calm down." Or, "He drew a smile on his picture of himself on the potty. Isn't that super? I love it that he feels proud about what he's done!"

Hence the important question "What stays the same over time?" cannot be answered fully without details about children's emotional lives. We may know that a 3-year-old girl can alternate feet while climbing stairs, but this is not the same as knowing that she sings gaily as she does so, or stomps in anger over an insult incurred an hour ago, or has to be coaxed to come upstairs because the "bogey man" might be there.

Where could preschoolers' budding emotional skills possibly come from? What fuels the development of their unique profiles of emotional competence? Both interpersonal and intrapersonal contributors are important, no doubt. How do parents, other caregivers, siblings, and peers contribute to preschoolers' growing emotional competence and to individual differences among them in this competence? How do changes in other areas of children's development, such as cognition, fuel emotional competence?

## Intrapersonal Contributions

Preschoolers differ in their age-appropriate abilities to categorize complex elements, such as other people, and to take the perspective of these other persons. Differences in these abilities contribute to differences in expressiveness, understanding, and regulation of emotions. As language, self-concept, perspective taking, and a moral sense develop, for example, so do the experience, expression, and understanding of complex emotions, such as empathy, contempt, guilt, and shame.

*Jenny knows that her friend is afraid of climbing to the top of the jungle gym, even though it is Jenny's favorite activity on the playground. This knowledge of her friend's feelings moderates Jenny's behavior during play with her. The direction of this moderation is governed by other factors: If Jenny is kind, she avoids this activity when playing with her friend; if she is a bit more self-concerned, she teases and goads her.*

## Interpersonal Contributions

Although each child brings a particular set of abilities to his or her emotional life, other persons clearly play a role in the development of emotional competence. That is, interpersonal socialization factors also contribute in a major way to the development of individual differences in emotional competence. Children learn much from various socializing agents about the appropriate expression of emotions, the nature of emotional expressions and situations, means of coping with emotions, and even potential reactions to others' positive and negative emotions.

During this point in the lifespan, the foremost socializers are parents. Most preschoolers enjoy continued close contact with their parents during this time period, even as they move into peer relationships. Parental modeling, coaching, and contingent reactions to children's emotions contribute to the children's own patterns of expressiveness, understanding of emotion, and coping with their own emotions and those of others.

Parents' own patterns of expressiveness are reflected in their children's expressiveness. Even preschoolers themselves are aware of these associations. When asked to articulate how she feels when her mother is happy, a preschooler may assert, "I give Mommy a big hug!" Another child reflects on his angry father: "I hide from him, I go outside; I don't like him when he's mad." Furthermore, parents who talk about emotions and foster this ability in their children enable their children to express certain optimal patterns of emotions.

> *Ranjit's mother calmly discusses her son's anger over not being allowed to sample grapes freely from the produce aisle as they stroll through the grocery store. A few shoppers eye her skeptically. But as Ranjit grudgingly grumbles about his desires, he is learning to use words to communicate emotional needs, rather than launching into a full-blown tantrum.*

And parents' specific reactions to their children's emotions encourage or discourage certain patterns of expressiveness. In the example above, the mother's calm response fosters not only Ranjit's acceptance of his own anger, but also his modulation of its intensity.

These aspects of socialization also contribute to young children's understanding of emotions. Parents' talking about emotion-laden experiences in daily life, accepting and encouraging children's emotional expressiveness, and expressing predominantly positive emotions all promote children's emotion knowledge.

> *When Joanna's father discusses her feelings about the end of the preschool year–the joy of an upcoming trip to the beach, but the accompanying sadness about missing friends–the guidance is quite direct. If Joanna's parents accompany their emotion coaching with positive expressiveness and a readiness to cultivate her emotional life by reacting to her emotions in a helpful, accepting way, then she is even more motivated to tackle the thorny issues centering around emotion understanding.*

Last, it is likely that parents' own emotions, coaching, and reactions to children's emotions influence children's means of emotion regulation.

> *Watching his mother break out in tears for the third time that day, Larry witnesses one way to deal with situations that require emotion regulation– just vent them! But he does not get to talk to his mother much about feelings, because she is too busy "letting out her anger." Perhaps the only message he does get is when his mother justifies her outbursts. The mother's scathing reactions to Larry's own emotions lead him to suppress his expressiveness, at least when she is present.*

Other socializers' contributions to emotional competence are also important. Peers and siblings can be very effective socializers of emotion. Their socialization is likely to differ substantially from that of parents, however: If a younger sibling becomes angry in a grocery store, the older sibling is not likely to be as patient and accepting as Ranjit's mother in the example above—answering anger, ridicule, or even desertion is far more probable! Obviously, the preschooler in question could deduce from these reactions that some people do *not* tolerate his anger—an equally important lesson.

## THE COMPLEX LINKAGE BETWEEN EMOTIONAL AND SOCIAL COMPETENCE

It is one thing to understand that children show differing patterns of emotional competence across ages and individuals. It is quite another matter to realize that these differences have a very real impact on how children work and play together, and on their feelings of mastery. Not only must parents, educators, and psychologists know what to look for in terms of young children's emotional development; they must know why such development is so crucial, and what aspects of it need fostering.

Successfully moving into the world of peers is a major developmental task of this period (Parker & Gottman, 1989; Waters & Sroufe, 1983). Young children's emotional competence—in particular, managing the emotional arousal that accompanies social interactions—is fundamental for this growing ability to interact and form relationships with others (Saarni, 1990). As Saarni (1990) states, "we are talking about how [children] can respond emotionally, yet simultaneously and strategically apply their knowledge about emotions and their expression to relationships with others, so that they can negotiate interpersonal exchanges and regulate their emotional experiences as well" (p. 116).

Joey, our "pirate" friend, uses emotion understanding, expressiveness, and regulation at full capacity during his play with peers, and this makes him a super playmate—he is more often part of peers' plans, is better liked, and has more friends than other children. So, to maximize social competence, researchers and others must carefully scrutinize how emotional competence allows a child to mobilize personal and environmental resources within peer interactions.

More specifically, if a young child shows certain patterns of expressiveness, he or she is more likely to be prosocial. A child who is sad or angry—either sitting on the sidelines of the group or querulously huffing around the room—is less likely to be able to see, let alone tend to, the emotional needs of others. Young children's own expressed emotions are also related to evaluations of their social competence made by important persons in their widening world: Happier children fare well, and angrier children worse.

Young children who understand emotion better also have more positive peer relations. The youngster who understands the emotions of others should interact more successfully when a friend gets angry with him or her, and the preschooler who can talk about his or her own emotions is also better able to negotiate disputes with friends.

> *If Matthew really wants the toy Jesse is holding, and is becoming increasingly frustrated, he will be most successful at getting what he wants if he tells his teacher, "Jesse is making me mad. Put on the timer so we'll know when it's my turn." Matthew probably also has more friends than he would if he progressed through his day grabbing and hitting when angry.*

Or, if a preschooler sees a peer bickering with another friend and correctly deduces the peer's sadness, she comforts her friend rather than retreating or even entering the fray. These accurate perceptions of emotion help children to react appropriately, thus bolstering their relationships. Learning to get along in groups of agemates also presses the preschool child toward regulating emotional expressiveness. When a preschooler begins to regulate his or her own emotions, he or she gets along more successfully with peers. In the example above, Matthew regulates his anger, and Jesse is glad that he does!

Intra- and interpersonal contributions to the important dimensions of emotional competence, and the contributions of emotional competence to social competence, form the foundation of a developmental model. I argue that both intrapersonal factors and interpersonal socialization of emotion within the preschool period contribute to the young child's understanding and regulation of emotions (i.e., expression of and reaction to emotions), and that these elements of emotional competence contribute to indices of social competence (see Figure 1.2). This model is a guiding framework throughout the book.

## DISTURBANCES IN THE DEVELOPMENT
## OF EMOTIONAL COMPETENCE

But what happens when the development of emotional competence goes awry? It is well and good to study the emotional development of

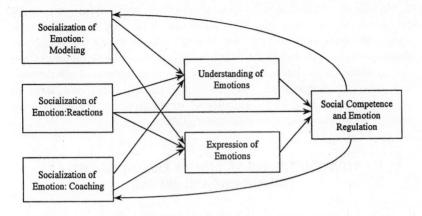

**FIGURE 1.2.** Developmental model of the socialization of emotional competence leading to social competence.

young children, as fascinating as it is, but what use can we make of this knowledge? An applied focus is an important foundation for this book.

Many societal problems with which communities struggle have strong emotional undercurrents. Often mental health difficulties are centered around deficits or unusual patterns of emotional expressiveness, understanding, and regulation. At the core of marital difficulties and child abuse lie anger, contempt, and shame. The experience of debilitating depression and anxiety is primarily emotional. On our highways and in our cities, images of anger predominate and too often blossom into violence.

To focus more specifically on childhood development, the lack of emotional competence is obviously central to intractable difficulties. Even a cursory review of the literature on behavior disorders reveals repeated mentions of emotional factors. Anger and other negative affect, as well as lack of positive affect or emotional support, are consistently described as characteristics of both children with behavior problems and their parents (Dadds, Sanders, Morrison, & Rebetz, 1992; Gardner, 1989). Moreover, such emotion-related behavioral characteristics often predict continuity in both externalizing and internalizing psychopathy (Werner, 1989). Thus, when developmental milestones of emotional competence are not negotiated successfully, preschoolers are at risk for psychopathology, both at the time and later in life (Zahn-Waxler, Iannotti, Cummings, & Denham, 1990).

To solve these pressing problems, emotional competence and the means to strengthen it must be addressed. Recognizing the importance of emotional competence in young children, and finding means of cultivating it, are essential for caregivers. Realizing when and how young children are at risk for delays, and learning to recognize disturbances in expected milestones of emotional competence, are equally important. Knowledge of risk factors, means of identifying delays in the development of emotional competence, and ways to intervene are vital, if the centrality of developing emotional competence is to be taken seriously (Knitzer, 1993).

## STUDYING THE YOUNG CHILD'S EMOTIONAL LIFE: THIS VOLUME AND BEYOND

If emotional competence is so very important, it behooves researchers, educators, and parents to understand what is really going on in the young child's emotional world. Ecologically valid measurement systems that require an investigator to enter a child's world, rather than vice versa, best allow researchers to discern young children's emotional competence. Thus, I argue forcefully—and attempt to illustrate amply throughout this book—that studies should be conducted within children's typical play activities. This can be accomplished by interacting with children one on one or by observing them. Ambiguous data or negative results may emanate from less sensitive modes of study.

How can we study emotional expressiveness and regulation—two important components of emotional competence? Fortunately, better operational definitions and other methodological advances have enabled successful examinations of children's emotional expressiveness patterns, whether these studies center on microanalytic, facial expressions of emotions or on more comprehensive, global indicators.

And how can we learn more about how preschoolers understand emotions? Asking young children to verbalize about issues of emotional competence leads directly to a quagmire of demand characteristics: A preschooler might think, "What does this man want me to do or say? How should I be feeling and acting in this setting?" Even more important, such means of questioning exist in a social vacuum (Saarni, 1987, 1990). A preschooler might query, "What is this lady talking about? Can I answer her at all? Why can't I just quit and go play?" New, ecologically valid means of examining understanding of emotion have also become available in response to these concerns.

Thus the stage is set for more fruitful inquiry into developmental change and individual differences in preschoolers' emotional competence. I attempt in this volume to give a picture of an exciting time—the unfolding of a vital set of emotional skills that sustain individuals' well-being and relationships. I intend to explore the very beginnings of these indispensable capacities to express, understand, and deal with the emotions of oneself and others. It is my hope to convey some of the energy inherent in these developments, and to inspire continued basic research into these engaging capabilities.

In subsequent chapters, then, I explore these important aspects of the changing emotional competencies of toddlers and preschoolers. First, in Chapter 2, I describe patterns and developments in children's emotional expressiveness—their consistent manner of showing emotions in various situations. I survey children's changing expression of the simplest, most basic emotions, which are separable according to facial, vocal, and behavioral indices; these include happiness, sadness, anger, and fear. Next I examine the emergence of more complicated emotions, which involve other people and self-consciousness, either implicitly or explicitly; these include shame, guilt, empathy, embarrassment, and pride. I also discuss children's increasing display of blended emotions, as well as their expanding demonstration of emotional display rules.

In Chapter 3, examining toddlers' and preschoolers' understanding of emotion, I take the view that young children are developing an impressive body of knowledge about both internal states and the causes of behavior (Wellman, 1990). Consequently, I explore their growing awareness of emotions in general and of specific discrete emotions. I describe toddlers' and preschoolers' abilities to use emotion labels, to recognize emotion situations, and to demonstrate knowledge of emotions' causes and consequences. Young children's use of emotion language within their families is also addressed. In addition, I describe the development of more complex aspects of understanding of emotion, such as knowledge of equivocal situations; conflicting expressive and situational cues; personalized experience of emotion; means of regulating both positive and negative emotions; display rules; and simultaneity and ambivalence. Adults also need to know what to expect in terms of preschoolers' understanding of their own and others' emotions. Finally, in both Chapters 2 and 3, I describe intrapersonal elements that are likely to contribute to individual differences in emotional competence during the preschool period.

Just as I describe typical developmental changes in aspects of emotional competence over the toddler and preschool period, I explore the roots of its individual differences. In Chapter 4, I review evidence of parents' influence on children's emotional expressiveness and understanding. Next, in Chapter 5, I explore new views of young children's ability to regulate their emotional expressiveness—what we know about developmental change and individual differences in emotion regulation, children's awareness of regulatory strategies, and socialization of emotion regulation during the preschool period. In Chapter 6, I focus on the social accomplishments supported by the young child's growing emotional competence.

I also hope to spotlight how essential these capabilities are to children's mental health, even at such an early age. If we have a clearer understanding of the roots of emotional competence, we will be better able to begin the vital task of facilitating it. So, in Chapter 7, I discuss young children who develop problems in emotional competence. Some deficits in emotional competence seem to reside in the children themselves. In contrast, other deficits in emotional competence seem to arise primarily from transactions with the environment. How can such children be identified? What can be done to assist them?

As concerned researchers, practitioners, and caregivers, we want to learn answers to these questions, so that we may help children develop optimal emotional skills. We are finally becoming aware of the importance of such emotional competence. We see that when children are not "smart" in this way, they are at long-term risk for depression; aggressiveness and violent crime; problems in marriage and parenting; and even poor physical health. As adults who care about children, we need to take emotional competence seriously. As Goleman (1995) put it so eloquently,

> [We must] make sure that every child is taught the essentials of handling anger or resolving conflicts positively . . . [we need to] teach empathy, impulse control, . . . [and] the fundamentals of emotional competence. By leaving the emotional lessons children learn to chance, we risk largely wasting the window of opportunity presented by the slow maturation of the brain to help children cultivate a healthy emotional repertoire. . . . In this sense, emotional [competence] goes hand in hand with education for character, for moral development, and for citizenship. (p. 286)

# ✵ Chapter 2

# Emotional Expressiveness

*E*xpressed emotions become ever more complex and elaborate during the toddler and preschool periods. Individual children differ in the intensity, frequency, and duration of their emotions; their own unique predominance of positive versus negative emotions; their use of pure versus mixed expressions; the speed with which they become emotional in a provocative situation; their level of understanding and attunement to others' emotions; and the time it takes them to resume their "even keel" (Hyson, 1994). These parameters of expression are important when one is trying to understand particular preschoolers and preschool emotional expressiveness in general. From my own work, many vivid examples come to mind.

## THE BALANCE OF POSITIVE AND NEGATIVE EMOTIONS

*Some children, like Juan, show predominantly positive emotions. He grins broadly the minute he sees a friend; when his teacher reads a funny passage of a book, he is delighted. If Juan were to cry, it is certain that his teachers would take him quite seriously. By contrast, Colin rarely shows positive emotions; he exhibits negative emotions or none at all. He is surly and combative with peers, and scowls during circle time, reacting negatively to the slightest innocent jostle from a neighbor. Everyone just tries to stay out of his way, and might not even notice a flicker of positivity*

19

*from him. But Zachary shows lots of both negative and positive emotions. He laughs uproariously on the playground when involved in rough-and-tumble play, but roars with anger when someone thwarts his building in the block corner. He keeps peers and adults alike on their toes.*

### FREQUENCY OF SPECIFIC EMOTION DISPLAYS

*Sebi often looks sad as he enters his preschool classroom and during circle time—eyelids heavy, lips drooping. His classmates look sad much less frequently. In contrast, Elizabeth is notable for sucking her thumb and shrinking back from the circle; on the playground she walks alone, and is startled when children run by vigorously. Her behaviors mark her frequent tension, seen only irregularly in her classmates.*

### INTENSITY OF EMOTION EXPRESSIONS

*Adults and peers need to be able to read children's expressiveness. Sometimes children's emotional intensity makes this easy; sometimes it is difficult, even when their frequency of expressiveness is relatively equal. On a bad day, Caroline's anger is explosive. She fusses and yells at people who make her mad; her wails are audible and her lashing out is visible across the large classroom. Davis, on the other hand, is expressive in a much more subtle, muted way. When he is annoyed, his lips purse slightly, his gaze is longer in duration, and his eyebrows lower a bit. Only a fairly attentive partner could pick up on this.*

### DURATION OF SPECIFIC EMOTIONS

*Midori's expressiveness flits from one emotion to another: One minute she is angry and struggling over a toy with a playmate, the next dissolving in laughter. Although her quick change disarms the dispute, sometimes it is hard to predict how interacting with her will turn out. But Roberto's style is different. He shows long periods of an equable but relatively neutral expression. When someone does something funny, though, he seems to retain the mood of delight and smiles for a long time. Similarly, he "holds onto" anger and grudges—even for days—when a friend does something mean. He is easier to predict than Midori is, but it is sometimes hard to break into his stable moods.*

### PURE VERSUS MIXED EMOTION EXPRESSIONS

*Children who show very blended expressions also take more effort to "read." Chelsea's vivid emotion displays vary between exceptionally clear depictions of joy and rage: She moves from a smile that lights up her entire visage to determined, fist-clenching, foot-stomping anger. But Elena's expressiveness is much more complicated to interpret, even for a trained observer. Elements of fear, pain, and joy play habitually on her face during social interactions when happiness, if anything, is most appropriate.*

SPEED OF EMOTION ONSET

*When someone crosses Taylor, his wrath is immediate. There is no question how he is feeling, no time to correct the situation before he erupts. Douglas, though, seems almost to consider the ongoing emotional situation. One can almost see annoyance building until he finally sputters, "Stop that!"*

I begin this chapter with an examination of what experiencing and expressing emotions mean to children and the people around them. I also highlight basic emotions' emergence and change across time. Most of the basic emotions emerge before a child is 2 years old. Personal emotional styles also become established early in the preschool period, adding to the complexity of expressiveness. Development of such personal styles adds new complexity to young children's emotional lives. Thus, I discuss this complexity and its stability across time and situations in young children's expressiveness.

The next major development in emotional expressiveness is the acquisition of social and self-conscious emotions, such as empathy, pride, guilt, embarrassment, and shame. I consider developmental trends in the expression of these emotions, and differentiate among the self-conscious emotions (i.e., pride, guilt, shame, and embarrassment). Subsequent developmental change in expressiveness includes the growing ability over the preschool period to manage emotional expression voluntarily, including posing expressions, showing expressiveness according to cultural display rules, and deception via hiding emotions. I address all these changes in expressive abilities in turn; they signal young children's increasing experience of a rich, complex emotional life, and their ability to modulate the expression of these emotions.

## EXPRESSION AND EXPERIENCE OF EMOTIONS ACROSS THE LIFESPAN

The patterns of expressiveness detailed in the examples above are important in determining whether a child is a good social partner— readable, predictable, and responsive. But the internal emotional experience of each preschooler is important, too. As clearly as these examples differentiate children according to parameters of expressiveness, emotion theorists still disagree about relation between early emotional expressiveness and emotional experience. As soon as infants exhibit the expressions associated with particular emotions, do they experience concomitant feelings? Do they experience them in the same general situations as older members of their cultures? Or are further cognitive development and socialization needed before toddlers and preschoolers can truly experience specifically discernible emotions? Izard (1991) favors the first view. In contrast, Lewis and colleagues (see, e.g., Lewis & Michalson, 1983) assert that other developments, especially the development of a sense of self, are necessary for the experience and meaningful expression of certain emotions. This argument is similar to the "Is cognition necessary for emotional experience?" question, addressed in Chapter 1.

In essence, the argument bears on whether expressed emotions, especially infants', are equivalent to a feeling state when no cognition occurs. In my view, this dispute often leads to a dead end in reasoning about children's emotions (see also Barrett, 1996). It is exceedingly difficult to access the feeling states of infants (and even those of toddlers and preschoolers, for that matter); their means of self-report are extremely limited. But remember that emotion can be experienced without cognitive appraisal, although appraisal often is necessary. My educated guess, then, is that although older persons have a powerful combination of emotional experience and understanding at their command, even young children are aware of, and certainly experience, some of the essential elements of emotions.

In other words, there is a "core of affective continuity" for experiencing each emotion—a specific and powerful constellation of vocal/facial/bodily expressions, behaviors, and associated meanings/goals/usefulness (however rudimentary) that is unique to each emotion (Campos & Barrett, 1984). An angry person, whether 3 years old or 30, lowers her voice almost to a growl, and glares, brows down, at the person or thing who made him or her mad. The person impatiently pushes at the doll's shoe that won't come off, or the ATM machine buttons that are not responding. The person consciously wants to *fix this problem,* and the anger helps to mobilize his or her efforts.

As the example of anger indicates, for the more basic emotions—happiness, sadness, anger, or fear—young children probably experience much the same feelings that their adult counterparts do in functionally equivalent situations. Consider also a case of fear in a child and adult:

*Leah feels afraid when asked to stand in front of a group of adults and recite a nursery rhyme. She wants to run out of the room, straight into the safety of her mother's arms. As a professor, her father has a similar affective experience each time he faces a new classroom full of students: He, too, wants to retreat into the safety of his wife's companionship.*

More complex emotions, such as shame, involve self-awareness, reflection, and evaluation; behavioral standards established by others; and the vicissitudes of experience. For such emotions, a child may feel the core of shame, but not the full range of shameful affect felt by an adult.

*If Leah begins to recite her rhyme, but forgets part of it, she may feel awful. The kernel of the feeling experience is there, and she wants to sink into the floor. In contrast, should her professor father forget a key element of his lecture, he feels foolish in front of a group of students who should admire him. Ashamed and embarrassed, he knows that his self-esteem has been dealt a blow.*

Yet the child and adult emotions have common themes: their expressive patterns, the behaviors associated with them, attempts to understand the causes of the emotion (in this case, shame), and decisions about future courses of action. So the expressed emotions have some experiential affective continuity, regardless of the time point in the lifespan at which they occur. And, again as asserted in Chapter 1, this emotional experience and expression impart functionally important sources of information to the child and others.

## INFORMATION IMPARTED BY EMOTIONAL EXPERIENCE AND EXPRESSION

Emotions are regulators of intra- and interpersonal behaviors: They let the person experiencing the emotions, and those nearby, know that "something must be done." This pragmatic view aids others' differentiation among expressions of early-emerging emotions, based on certain features (Barrett & Campos, 1991); it can assist children themselves in appreciating the uniqueness of their own emotional experiences.[1] Consequently, young children's expression and experience of emotions impart several important types of information.

1. *"What emotion is this?"* Emotions need to be identified by the child experiencing the emotion and by other people interacting with him or her. First, the basic emotions (e.g., happiness, sadness, anger, and fear) often have specific vocal qualities, intonation patterns, and

particular patterns of facial movement (Izard, Dougherty, & Hembree, 1980; but see Russell, 1994). These are important signals both to the child experiencing them and to other persons. Happiness is defined by a combination of smiles, laughter, and voices with "pearly," relaxed pitch. In contrast, sadness is marked by crying, inner corners of eyebrows lifted, corners of lips down, and slow, steady-pitched speech. Anger is seen in lowered brows, tense lower lips, and staring. The speech of angry persons is clipped, abrupt, and often loud. Tight brows, raised and drawn together, with high-pitched voice, indicate fear. Young children express and experience all these basic emotions, and begin to recognize their expressive patterns in themselves and others (see Chapter 3).

2. *"What should I do now?"/"What is he or she likely to do now?"* Emotions often lead to this second question, whether implicitly or explicitly. A number of theorists suggest that different emotions have particular action tendencies associated with them: fleeing with fear, aggression with anger, withdrawal or tearfulness with sadness. In general, young children develop common action tendencies for differing emotions. Fortunately, many adults are correct when they use these action tendencies to identify young children's emotions.

3. *"Why is this emotion important to me/to the child experiencing it?"* Emotions have adaptive functions that serve as internal teaching mechanisms. They carry personal meaning for the child experiencing them. These adaptive functions can help them to differentiate emotions. For example, the adaptive function of disgust is protection of the self from noxious substances (e.g., the tasting of a rotten apple leads to future avoidance). In contrast, the adaptive function for fear is avoidance of dangerous situations. A 4-year-old boy experiences fear when he is at the top of the monkey bars at day care. He comes to understand that this feeling signals possible danger—"I am scared when I go a little too far"—and, ideally, he does something to become safer. Over time, young children also learn to better understand the experiential difference among emotions. Thus feelings of disgust are associated with getting away from "yucky" things, whereas feelings of fear are linked with avoiding danger.

Discerning the adaptive functions of a child's emotions also can be helpful for adults who are involved with children. What does this emotion mean *for the child*? Is the child who rejects an unfamiliar food experiencing disgust or simply being defiant? Seeing his son's fear on the monkey bars, the 4-year-old's father should at least consider whether the boy feels truly unsafe. Reflecting a moment about a child's previous experiences can help a caregiver understand what emotion is being experienced, and respond appropriately.[2]

4. *"What does this display of emotion communicate to people observing it?"* The child and observing adults also distinguish individual emotions while they are felt, based on what the feelings signify to others in the particular context. Feelings can be socially significant. When a 3-year-old girl's mother catches her playing when she's supposed to be sleeping, the girl experiences fear. Because the child gradually understands the social meaning of the parent's frown and sigh (a return to bed, and maybe even punishment, are imminent), her experience of emotion centers on the social significance of this behavior: "If I play around after bedtime, my parents will not like it. That makes me scared to sneak around."

Knowing the social significance of the expression or experience of emotion is important, because these vary for each emotion. A 5-year-old boy witnessing a peer crying when he stumbles in the hallway of their school shows disgust. He understands the social meaning of such a lapse in self-control, because he now knows the norms of his peer group and engages in social comparison: "Everyone will laugh. I say 'yuck!' "

5. *"What am I/What is the person experiencing the emotion trying to accomplish?"* Goals are very important in the experience of emotion. The work of Nancy Stein and her colleagues helps illuminate children's interpretations of the significance of emotions (e.g., Stein & Jewett, 1986; Stein & Levine, 1989, 1990; Stein & Trabasso, 1989). Stein posits that a complex process of understanding underlies emotional experience. Emotion is aroused when an event signals that something the individual wants, or does not want, is about to happen. Consider a 5-year-old girl whose drawing is destroyed by a peer. Her ongoing activity has been disrupted, and she tries to figure out what was happening. As she notices her problem, she also becomes aware of her arousal. She understands that something has happened that she doesn't want, and she feels her heart pumping in a surge of anger. An increase in heart rate is associated with arousal of an emotion.[3]

But individual goals are crucial in determining which emotion is experienced. Again, consider the child creating a drawing. She's totally absorbed in her activity. A playmate comes over and deliberately knocks her arm, hard. The emotional result of this peer's actions could conceivably be either anger or sadness. The emotion that the girl experiences depends on the lens through which she views the event—that of the peer's provocative act, or the loss of the drawing. Is it her goal to conserve something she has created with her own hands? Is she sad over the injury to something personal? Or is she more concerned with the goal of her relationship with her friend, and therefore angry that he did something mean?

Further examples will serve to clarify this integrated perspective. A 4-year-old girl sees a big, friendly dog. After encountering this event, she encodes it in her memory and tries to understand it. Aspects either of the external environment (e.g., the actual approach of the dog), or of internal processing (e.g., an earlier encounter with a dog) can cause emotional events. These patterns of understandings can lead to two possible emotions. If the child focuses on the dog's happy "grin," she concludes, "Something new is happening, and it will be something I like"; she feels happiness. She realizes that the goal of having "a fun time" may be realized, and approaches the dog. In contrast, if the child focuses on the dog's big, open mouth, she thinks, "Something new is impending, and it will be something I don't like"; she feels fear. In this case, the child clings to her mother or runs away.

Either way, the child is aware of valuable emotional information: (a) the change in a valued state ("something I like or don't like"); (b) the conditions that caused the change; (c) the consequences of the change for goal maintenance or attainment; and (d) plans for maintaining, reinstating, or abandoning a goal. These understandings increasingly influence which specific emotion the child detects (see also Fischer et al., 1989). To illustrate, a pattern of understandings for sadness is "wanting but not having something," as when a parent departs; plans include searching for the parent or using a substitute caregiver for comfort. A pattern of understandings for anger is "not wanting but having an event," as when a peer takes away a toy; plans include getting the toy back through whatever means necessary.

Over time, the orderly pattern of these emotional experiences related to certain goals in specific eliciting situations helps the child to discern the general differences among discrete emotions (see Chapter 3). A child also comes to make plans based upon this experience of emotions, and to manage emotions in increasingly organized ways (see Chapter 5).

## BASIC EMOTIONS: CHANGE ACROSS TIME

By the time children reach their third year, they are experiencing and expressing a variety of emotions. Their emotion repertoires include all the basic emotions—joy, sadness, anger, fear, interest—and the way emotions are expressed are increasingly differentiated. Preschoolers can share positive emotions together, but they can also share negative emotions:

*Micah squeals in anger when his garage of blocks falls apart. He thinks, correctly, that Lan made it fall. Lan says he'll help build it up again, but then backs off, looking sad. Micah screams at Lan again; Lan backs away, still sad and whining. Jamell joins the fray, angrily defending Micah.*

Malatesta and colleagues investigated changes in such patterns of emotional expressiveness between infancy and 3 years of age (Malatesta, Culver, Tesman, & Shepard, 1989; see also Fogel & Reimers's [1989] commentary on this work). These researchers expected facial displays of emotion to decrease in frequency during the period, if young children were learning to curtail expressiveness according to the display rules of our culture. In contrast, they expected vocal expressiveness to stay stable, because vocal expressiveness is relatively difficult to control. But, contrary to expectations, toddlers' total vocal emotional expressiveness actually increased from the second to the third year. There was essentially no change in facial expressiveness. What sense could be made of these unexpected outcomes? Apparently display rule usage comes later (see below), and linguistic output makes the vocal channel even more attractive as an eloquent conveyor of emotional meaning.

Malatesta and colleagues also examined changes at the level of individual emotions. Both verbal and vocal expressions of joy, interest, surprise, and anger increased. Vocal expressions of sadness decreased, while facial expressiveness of this emotion remained the same. Hence, children remain emotionally intense early in the preschool period, with both facial and vocal channels serving to clearly communicate emotion. They do not yet limit their overall emotional expressiveness.

Nonetheless, these data allow for several extrapolations about the emotional expressiveness of young children in naturalistic situations. By 3 years of age, children are able to alternate or exchange modes of expressiveness as the situation demands, as well as to inhibit or intensify expressiveness as needed. Context becomes more important as a determinant of the type of emotional expressiveness. For instance, glaring angrily at a peer during play is more appropriate, and more effective, than screaming and attracting unwanted maternal attention; by contrast, a vocal signal of distress is more appropriate than a visual one when a child falls down in the yard and needs a parent to come and help (see "Control of Expressiveness and Adherence to Display Rules," below).

Expression of some emotions also becomes more frequent than others. In peer settings, for example, happiness and anger are expressed more often than either sadness or pain and distress (Denham,

1986; Fabes, Eisenberg, Nyman, & Michealieu, 1991). Fortunately, as relieved parents and caregivers can attest, negativity decreases for most children as they move into the preschool period (Cole, Michel, & Teti, 1994; Kopp, 1994). Blended emotions also appear (Cole, 1985; Izard, 1991). Boys engaged in rough-and-tumble play can show clear signs of both happiness and anger at the same time. Blended emotions can confound adults, who ask themselves whether children need assistance or are merely having fun.

Sex differences in the expression of emotion have been noted during this period among preschoolers. These sex differences usually parallel differences in problematic emotions reported for boys and girls at later ages. Fabes et al. (1991) reported that preschool boys expressed more anger than girls. In contrast, girls expressed more sadness. Malatesta-Magai et al. (1994) also found similar early sex differences in expressiveness.

In short, overall emotion expression does not diminish over time early in the preschool period; rather, it is transformed, becoming more flexible, complex, and differentiated (Malatesta et al., 1989). The subtlety and complexity of emotional expression continue to increase markedly throughout the preschool years. Increased ability to think and solve problems supports these systematic changes in the breadth and complexity of preschoolers' emotionality (Barrett & Campos, 1991). The number and variety of interactions that the child can appreciate as significant, the variety of means by which the child can enact an action tendency, and the child's ability to modulate emotional reactions are all related to cognitive development.

## INDIVIDUAL DIFFERENCES IN BASIC EMOTIONS: STABILITY ACROSS TIME

Developmental changes in children's emotional expressiveness is accompanied by increasingly stable patterns of expressiveness for individual children. In other words, children tend to have distinguishable emotional styles, and these styles show stability across time. Parents and teachers talk about children as if this were the case; they exclaim over one child's "sunny personality" and another's constant outbursts of anger over both small and large events.

Stable individual differences in enduring patterns of expressiveness are indeed apparent by 2 years of age (e.g., in irritability; see Riese, 1990; Vaughn, Contreras, & Seifer, 1993). In their work, Malatesta et al. (1989) documented the facial expressions of children's basic emotions in several contexts across the first 22 months of life. These researchers reported that "children tend to show continuity in their emotional expressive patterns across a range of discrete emotions and signals" (p. 61). In accord with Riese's data, only negative emotional expressions—sadness, anger, knit brow, and pressed lips—showed stability. Sadness and anger at 7 months best predicted sadness and anger at 22 months.

My colleagues and I also examined the stability of patterns of emotional expressiveness across the first 30 months of life (Denham, Lehman, Moser, & Reeves, 1995), although our methodology differed somewhat from that of Malatesta et al. and of Riese. Our results indicated that the nature of emotional expressions of anger, fearfulness, interest, and joy often showed between-age stability at six measurement points between 6 weeks and 30 months. Data from LaFreniere and Sroufe (1985) extended stability findings to the later preschool years: The positive and negative expressiveness of 4- and 5-year-olds showed cross-time and cross-context stability.

Taken together, these studies demonstrated clear individual differences in infants', toddlers', and preschoolers' expressive patterns, with several emotions showing significant cross-time stability over several assessments during the infant–preschool agespan. What explanations can be put forward for such stability—for the emergence of such emotional styles? Expressive patterns, though flexible, can become relatively ingrained, stable components of personality (Malatesta et al., 1989; see also Tomkins, 1962, 1963, 1991). Certain children are aroused particularly easily, or aroused by certain stimuli, perhaps through genetic pathways. Another reason for emotional styles is the possibility that children acquire ways of construing the events in their world, or schemas for interpreting potentially emotional events. Malatesta and colleagues argue that negative expressive patterns become habitual more readily than positive patterns do.

Despite researchers' reports that individual differences in emotional expressions are stable, it is important to note that the stability coefficients in studies are relatively low, lower than those for mothers across the same general time period (Malatesta et al., 1989). So, although young children's emotional expressiveness may be partially biologically based, it is also subject to effects of enculturation, learning, and context.

Why are these developments in the area of expressiveness important? Adults can find it useful to recognize these developments in discerning what stays the same and what changes across this agespan, for children in general and for a particular child. It is worthwhile to pinpoint individual differences in the development of expressiveness; differing patterns of emotionality contribute to a child's relative ability to get along with others and become involved productively in the world. Knowing about particular preschoolers' personal styles and the increasing sophistication of their emotional worlds can also help adults to live with them more peacefully and fruitfully. Caregivers, parents, and early childhood educators are better informed when they know the normal developments in preschoolers' expressive patterns. Such information helps them cope well with children's strengths and weaknesses in this important area.

## THE DEVELOPING EXPERIENCE AND EXPRESSION OF SELF-CONSCIOUS AND SOCIAL EMOTIONS

The flexibility, modulation, and increased complexity in the expression of basic emotions go along with the appearance of social and self-conscious emotions in a preschooler's expressive repertoire. These emotions include empathy, pride, guilt, shame, embarrassment, envy, and contempt. The relatively simple patterns of understandings that accompany the basic emotions must be elaborated so that the child experiences these more complex emotions. Both cognitive development and specific socialization experiences allow for this elaboration.

> *Joelle knows that it is not okay to break her mom's ceramic figurine, and looks around furtively as she tries to forces the pieces back together.*

> *Ben sees his friend Joshua wet his pants, and knowing this defies social convention, sneers. Joshua just wants to sink into the ground.*

### Cognitive Foundations

Self-recognition and self–other differentiation develop through the second year of life and are foundations for the expression of certain emotions (Lewis, 1993a; Zahn-Waxler & Radke-Yarrow, 1990). These ideas allow young children to experience and express self-conscious and social emotions. As toddlers begin to rely on representational thought and the use of symbols, they realize that they are distinctly separate from others. This distinctive self-awareness is necessary for the experience and expression of embarrassment, empathy, and envy (Lewis, 1993a). In addition, young children come to recognize their own success or failure at day-to-day tasks. Both self-awareness and an understanding of standards and rules are necessary for the experience and expression of pride, shame, and guilt. Toddlers who understand that an object is flawed, or that a standard has been breached, demonstrate a nascent form of guilt by offering apologies and showing visible distress (Kochanska, Casey, & Fukumoto, 1995).

So even very young children actively interpret the arousal attendant upon success, failure, or wrongdoing. Preschoolers may experience shame, guilt, pride, empathy, and embarrassment according to specific patterns of understanding about their goals (cf. Stein & Levine's [1989, 1990] focus only on basic emotions). For example, shame may be characterized by this interpretation: "I've done something [the novel event that leads to emotional arousal] that decreases the likelihood that I can continue to feel good about myself. I have experienced this event and this feeling; I don't want them to continue, but it's overwhelming. I'd better hide [or lash out, etc.]." The interpretation for pride may be the obverse of this event analysis (see also Chapter 3). The experience and expression of guilt, in contrast, might include the following interpretation: "I've done something [again, the novel event] that makes it unlikely that other people will continue to be happy with me. I have experienced this event and feeling, but don't want it to continue. I'd better make amends in some way." The experience and expression of empathy can similarly be mapped out according to an event analysis: "Something has happened to someone else, and this event decreases the likelihood of good feelings for them and for me. I have vicariously experienced this event and feeling, and don't want them to continue. I'd better help the person [or leave the scene to lessen my own arousal]."

Clearly, very specific cognitive attainments of self-understanding and rule internalization, as well as increased ability to perform the social-cognitive event analyses above, are central to preschoolers' new experience and expression of social and self-conscious emotions. One key way that children come to structure these cognitive interpretations of their emotional arousal as self-conscious or social emotions is no doubt via internalization of socialization messages from the adults in their world.

## Socialization Foundations

In concert with these cognitive foundations, socialization contributes to individual differences in the experience and expression of such emotions as empathy, pride, guilt, shame, embarrassment, envy, and contempt (Lewis, 1993a). Socializers' messages clarify for a child the very nature of success, failure, and wrongdoing. Parents react very clearly with emotional, behavioral, and linguistic messages about the child's adherence to the family's standards, rules, and goals (Lewis, 1993a). They also comment explicitly about the child's competence across a range of domains.

So parents' reactions to children's success, failure, and wrongdoing figure largely in which events each child considers noteworthy and emotionally arousing. This explicit content of standards and rules is communicated by parents. Some parents may expect children not to touch fragile bric-a-brac. The preschooler who does so despite this implicit rule experiences a parent's scowling face, a loud "No!" or even a slap, and perhaps a statement such as "Why can't you ever listen?" Or consider a young girl exploring in a pile of dirt with her teddy bear. She is met with a cold, abrupt removal to the bathtub, and with the parent's contemptuous words, "Only you can find so many ways to get into trouble!" Similarly, a boy who plays Power Ranger on his mother's new sideboard, deeply scratching it, is promptly reminded of the house rule that "it is not okay to climb on furniture."

In addition, much information about achievement is given by parents. For example, some families value early preacademic performance. When a preschooler in such a family learns to write his or her name, the child is rewarded with a parent's broad smile, a delighted hug, and a statement such as "That's super! I knew you could do it!" Finally, the vicarious experience of the others' emotions can also be fueled by parents. Young preschoolers just learning to move around skillfully in their play environment—and only beginning to interact purposively with peers—may be told, "It really, really hurts Johnny when you knock him down like that."

Such socializing discourse not only imparts emotional meaning to everyday events, but also fuels the ways children "figure out" how to feel. Feelings of shame are natural outcomes when parents focus on a child's inadequacy and are unclear about the exact nature of the transgression. In contrast, the child playing Power Ranger on the sideboard feels guilt because his mother has focused only on the importance of not breaking rules, without accompanying contempt.

In short, socialization practices specific to early transgressions, failures, and successes affect the development of a child's tendency to feel and express complex self-conscious and social emotions. Such experiences are implicit in the following descriptions of empathy, pride, guilt, shame, and embarrassment (see also Chapter 4). For each of these emotions, I describe means of expression, developmental change during the preschool period, and contextual parameters important to its expression.

## A SOCIAL EMOTION: EMPATHY

Empathy, the ability to feel the emotions of another, is thought to motivate caring and concerned actions toward other persons in need. It is a social, not a self-conscious, emotion. Preschool-age children can feel empathy; they can show it with their expressions, their words, and their actions. A mother and child are conversing:

MOTHER: I'm kind of feeling sad.

CHILD: Don't feel sad. I'm your friend (*patting the mother, wiping her tears away, and hugging her*). Don't cry.

These prosocial behaviors can emanate from a visceral understanding of the mother's plight, from the experience of empathy.

There has been much debate regarding the precise definition of empathy, ways to measure it, and its likely correlates, especially in children (e.g., Lennon & Eisenberg, 1987). Some of these problems might be eased by a functionalist analysis of emotion. First, what kind of emotional arousal occurs when a child sees another person in distress? How can we distinguish children's empathy, know it when we see it? Second, what action tendencies are associated with empathy? Third, what are the likely goals of the child experiencing empathy?

Guided by these functionalist questions, researchers have made a useful distinction between two types of empathic responses: sympathetic reactions to another person's distress and personal distress reactions (Batson, 1991; Eisenberg, Schaller, et al., 1988). The facial muscle and physiological indices of these two patterns differ. Sympathetic expressions include knit brows, slightly open mouth, and heart rate deceleration (suggestive of concentration). In contrast, distress expressions are indexed by indrawn, raised brows, licking of lips or touching of the face, and heart rate acceleration (often found in fear). Children who experience sympathy are likely to behave prosocially, but those who experience personal distress more often act distressed themselves. So, in both sympathy and personal distress, there is an empathic component: Another's distress has aroused the child's vicarious emotion and associated action tendencies. But the child's construal of his or her own goals is central to the distinction. Focus on the other leads to a sympathetic reaction, and focus on one's own predicament leads to a personal distress reaction.

Both social-psychological and behavioral-genetic studies lend credence to the differentiation of these two types of empathic responses. The tendency to react either sympathetically or with distress to others' distress has a genetic component (Zahn-Waxler, Robinson, & Emde, 1992). These researchers found that identical twins were more similar in empathic style, whether sympathetic or reflecting personal distress, than were fraternal twins. It is likely, then, that the observable differences between the two types of empathic response arise from differing patterns of biological arousal, although focusing on the self or the other is no doubt also important. Hence children's empathic reactions are sometimes predominantly sympathetic, whereas at other times they are more indicative of personal distress. Both developmental and individual differences in these aspects of empathy are evident.

## Developmental Change in Preschoolers' Empathy

In terms of the developmental progression of empathy, children as young as 2 years of age are able to broadly interpret others' emotional states, experience these feeling states in response to others' predicament, and attempt to alleviate discomfort in others (Zahn-Waxler & Radke-Yarrow, 1982, 1990). Very young children sometimes evidence sympathetic concern and attempts at active aid. A 2-year-old boy attempted to soothe his older brother with a multifaceted calming campaign (Goleman, 1995). The younger child implored his brother to stop crying, beseeched his mother to help, adopted a mothering mode himself, tried to lend a pragmatic helping hand in putting away Lego blocks, and distracted him with a toy car. Only when these efforts failed did the 2-year-old give up on caring and kindness, and adopt his mother's no-nonsense style: "Stop crying . . . Smack your bottom!" (Dunn, 1988, pp. 94–95).

Many, though obviously not all, of this 2-year-old's efforts were sympathetic. But some very young children have not yet developed the capacity to experience fully the complex emotion of empathy:

> *Alberta was hurt on the playground. Mark began to cry, too, although he had nothing to do with the event. Belinda just looked at Alberta as she cried–maybe to see what was the matter–but she showed no emotional arousal.*

So expressions of sympathy and the control of personal distress continue to change across the preschool period.

Evidence of more sophisticated indicators of empathy is associated with self-recognition. Children who are old enough to have attained a stable notion of the self–other distinction are more likely to show a sympathetic reaction to another's condition (Bischof-Kohler, 1988; Zahn-Waxler & Radke-Yarrow, 1990). Accordingly, there is empirical evidence that the frequency of sympathetic concern increases with age.

Personal distress also decreases as children mature. Nonetheless, personal distress in response to others' emotions can still be evoked; for instance, consider the stilling of motor activity and facial signs of worry when a young preschooler is trapped with quarreling parents.

And, despite the age-related decrease, preschoolers still show personal distress more than older children. In response to films of persons in difficult circumstances, preschoolers express more fear than either sadness or concern (Strayer, 1993; Wilson & Cantor, 1985). Grade-school-age children show more concern than sadness or fear—an opposite pattern of responses. The preschoolers seem less reactive emotionally to the televised characters' dilemmas and fears than to the fear-provoking stimulus itself. This lack of sympathy is not due to the younger children's inability to recognize the televised characters' emotion; rather, their own personal distress gets in the way. The scary element of films such as those in these studies is more powerful for them than the plight of the story's main character.

Other investigators have focused on developmental change in the action tendencies associated with empathy—behavioral, rather than facial, indicators. Here again even the youngest preschoolers are capable of showing early forms of sympathy and personal distress. Two-year-olds show anxious/worried and concerned *behaviors* in response to another's predicament, including freezing (not moving) and just looking, as well as early, sometimes clumsy, attempts at active aid (Zahn-Waxler & Radke-Yarrow, 1982).

Behavioral reactions to peers' crying have been tracked extensively across the preschool age period. Phinney, Feshbach, and Farver (1986) studied 28- to 48-month-olds' responses to crying peers over 290 crying episodes. The relative frequency of positive reactions to crying peers was 2.1 per hour, with older preschoolers responding sympathetically more often to crying peers than younger children. Similarly, Kiselica and Levin (1987) observed preschoolers and found that sympathetic/empathic reactions occurred at a rate of 1.6 per hour. Two-year-olds mostly showed sustained attention to a peer's crying, with 3-year-olds in transition to empathic intervention. The 4- and 5-year-olds most often showed empathic concern, as evidenced by comforting their friends. Thus, behavioral indicators of sympathy, like facial ones, increase with age across the preschool period.

In general, then, both facial and behavioral indicators of sympathy increase during the preschool period, and personal distress reactions decrease but are still common. Despite these age trends, individual children also show distinct inclinations toward one pattern of empathy or the other.

## Individual Differences in Young Children's Empathy

Children often show a predominance of either sympathetic or personal distress empathy. One way of pinpointing these personal empathic styles is to examine their correlates. Because they focus on the distress of the other, sympathetic reactions should be more conducive than personal distress reactions to positive social behavior. This pattern has been found in a number of studies, in which preschoolers who showed indices of concern behaved more prosocially than those who showed personal distress, to both televised and "live" victims of distress (Eisenberg et al., 1990; Eisenberg, McCreath, & Ahn, 1988; Mason, Mitchell-Copeland, & Denham, 1996).

But, although these styles of reacting to others' emotions are often inversely related, this is not a necessary condition (Zahn-Waxler & Radke-Yarrow, 1990); a child can be both sympathetic and distressed at the intensity of another's distress. The 3-year-old daughter of a depressed parent may treat her crying mother very tenderly, almost assuming the role of caregiver, but may also feel quite a bit of distress herself. Conversely, a child may also be relatively oblivious to other persons' emotions, or may react in an emotionally anomalous manner, neither sympathetic nor distressed:

> Michael continued quiet solitary play with his truck, despite a furious argument ensuing in one corner of the sandbox, and the glee of two children chasing each other nearby. Another day, he actually laughed when Jamila was hurt.

## Moderators of the Experience of Empathy

So any given child may be high on both sympathy and personal distress, may be low on both, or may show a particularly distinctive type of either sympathetic or personal distress. But other extenuating factors may moderate such personal styles. Several parameters of a sympathy-provoking experience, as well as personal attributes, have been posited as important in determining young children's empathic responsiveness.

### Similarity to the Victim and Focus of Attention

Children can evidence either sympathy or distress reactions, or no emotional arousal, depending upon the situation in which they find themselves. Preschoolers tend to show more sympathy when the distressed person is similar to them in some way (or they are at least familiar with the other's experience), or when they focus on the other's emotional neediness.

In particular, seeing the person experiencing distress as like oneself can be important in motivating sympathy or personal distress. M. A. Barnett (1984) told preschool-age subjects that they had failed or succeeded at either a puzzle board or a ball-pitch game; others were allowed merely to observe the game. After either participating or watching the tasks, children then watched a videotaped vignette of another child failing the ball-pitch game. Thus, the similarity or dissimilarity of the subjects' experience on a familiar or unfamiliar game was varied systematically (see Table 2.1). Young children's sympathy to an unhappy agemate was enhanced when an observing child had a similar unpleasant experience and could say, "I know how you feel." In particular, children who had failed at the ball-pitch game showed more concern and rated their own mood as less positive when seeing another child in difficulty with the same game.

Although similarity with the other's situation generally enhances sympathy, the story is more complicated than this. Given the similarity of shared experience, children's locus of attention is also important.

> *Five-year-old Jason feels strong emotions while watching Andrew being spanked by his mother. Depending on the situation and his focus, he feels intense sympathy for Andrew or sees Andrew's situation as a portent of his own distress. If Andrew has misbehaved before Jason arrives (e.g., his mother has just discovered Play-Doh in the VCR), Jason sees the distress Andrew is feeling, focuses on his friend's pitiful tears, and feels sympathy. In contrast, if both boys have conspired to transfer much of the sandbox's contents to the flower beds, Jason witnesses Andrew's tears, thinks that his turn for spanking is next, and experiences much personal distress.*

Similarly, when children see another child in a predicament, those who have been induced to focus on that child's dilemma show more sympathy than children who are induced to consider their own sadness (Barnett, Howard, & Melton, 1982; see also Barnett, King, Howard, & Dino, 1980).

## Gender and General Context

Gender of the victim and context of distress also moderate sympathetic behavioral reactions to distress. In at least one study, preschoolers were more likely to console crying girls, and criticize crying boys (Phinney et al., 1986). Thus, children behaved in accordance with gender stereotypes of emotion at a young age! And although children were lone observers only 19% of the times they saw others crying, they were more positive and prosocial when the peer cried alone than when in interaction with others. Furthermore, a friend's crying elicits more sympathetic behavior than a mere acquaintance's (Costin & Jones, 1992; Farver & Branstetter, 1994). Being confronted with a lone other's, or a friend's, distress evokes social norms and increases one's feelings of responsibility, even at a very early age.

### Emotionality and Personal Emotional Profile

Children's emotional expressiveness also moderates empathic responsiveness to others' emotions. That is, children need to be emotionally secure, and to have experience with emotions themselves, to be sympathetically responsive to others (Strayer, 1980; Denham, 1986).

Feeling generally positive emotions oneself makes it easier to focus on others' emotions. Along these lines, children with more positive temperaments and more positive peer interactions are more likely to exhibit behavioral sympathy to a crying peer (e.g., comforting, mediating; Farver & Branstetter, 1994). In my work, I have found that preschoolers who are more often happy react more sympathetically to the negative affect of their peers (Denham, 1986). Lennon and Eisenberg (1987) have gone one step further: They have demonstrated that preschoolers' happy displays evidenced *during* prosocial behaviors are related to the frequency of their unrequested prosocial behavior. Therefore, not only does feeling happier most of the time promote sympathy; even more pointedly, so does feeling good when prosocial behavior is called for.

Several theories of empathy and sympathy also predict that negative affect, rendering the child more self-focused, hampers the ability to respond prosocially (Eisenberg, 1986). I have found just such a pattern: Children who are generally angrier or sadder respond less sympathetically to peers' distress than do those who are more often happy (Denham, 1986; see also Strayer, 1993).

Overall emotionality also allows young children to recognize others' feelings, and thus to empathize with them. Children exhibiting higher overall emotionality, measured in number of displays per minute, are more likely to respond sympathetically to peers' emotions. They more often match happy displays, leave the area of angry displays, and/or reinforce, help, share, or comfort in response to peers' emotions (Denham, 1986). Thus, experiencing a variety of mostly positive,

**TABLE 2.1.** Amount of Sympathy Shown to Videotaped Peer

| Game played by child | Outcome experienced by child | |
|---|---|---|
| | Same as protagonist | Different from protagonist |
| Same as protagonist | +++ | 0 |
| Different from protagonist | + | − |

*Note.* Data from M. A. Barnett (1984).

moderate-intensity emotions should facilitate sympathetic reactions to others' emotions (Hoffman, 1984; Strayer, 1980).

## Understanding of Emotions

Understanding the emotions that are being displayed by others is an important substrate for responding empathically. Certainly, knowing whether another child is in pain, sad, angry, disgusted, or even contemptuous makes a big difference in how one responds. I have shown that children with higher-level emotion knowledge are less apt to merely ignore their parents' emotions. Children who are more capable of explaining emotions in conversations with parents are also more sympathetic in response to peers' emotions (Denham, Renwick-DeBardi, & Hewes, 1994). Finally, understanding of emotions contributes to children's sympathetic responsiveness in structured situations with an adult (Denham, 1986; Denham & Couchoud, 1991).

## Summary

Sympathetic reactions to the distress of others increase across the preschool period. Personal distress does not disappear as children become capable of sympathy. Both facial and behavioral indices of sympathy appear, and are moderated by such factors as gender, self-focus, context of the other's distress, similarity to the distressed person, and familiarity with the distressing experience. Other elements of the child's emotional expressiveness, as well as understanding of emotions, figure importantly in empathic responsiveness.

## SELF-CONSCIOUS EMOTIONS: GUILT, SHAME, PRIDE, AND EMBARRASSMENT

### Differentiating among Self-Conscious Emotions

Self-conscious emotions also emerge during toddlerhood and the preschool years. Shame and guilt reactions are often correlated and share critical defining features, including self-consciousness, self-evaluation, internal attribution, moral overtones, and interpersonal jeopardy concerns (Ferguson & Stegge, 1995). Because of these shared features, some investigators continue to lump guilt, shame, and even embarrassment into one "feeling-bad-about-performance" emotion, as contrasted to pride, the "feeling-good-about-performance" emotion.

But research repeatedly underscores the unique functional aspects of the self-conscious emotions of shame and guilt (Tangney, 1990, 1991; Tangney, Flicker, Barlow, & Miller, 1996). In guilt, the key concern is with a particular behavior. Guilt involves a feeling that "I *did* that horrible *thing*." Children and adults experiencing guilt often report a nagging concentration on the specific transgression—thinking of it over and over, wishing they had behaved differently or could undo the bad deed.

Feelings of shame also can arise from a specific behavior or transgression. But the ramifications of shame extend well beyond those of guilt (Lewis, 1992). The "bad behavior" is not seen as needing a simple reparation or apology; in fact, a reparation may not even be sufficient to assuage this feeling. Rather, the offensive behavior is seen as a reflection of an equally offensive self.

Thus, the key concern when feeling shame is with one's worth as a person. Shame involves a feeling that "*I* am an unworthy, bad person." People in the midst of a shame experience often report a sense of shrinking, of "being small." They feel worthless, powerless, and exposed. Although shame does not necessarily involve an actual observing audience, one often imagines how one's defective self would appear to others. Because of this feeling of exposure, shame often motivates avoidance. Shame is generally more painful than guilt; consequently, people feeling shame often report a desire to flee from the shame-inducing situation, to "sink into the floor and disappear." And this discomfort can be lasting: The little girl who journeys into the dirt pile with her teddy bear may remember her shame even years later.

Affective styles of more often feeling ashamed or guilty are well established by middle childhood (Tangney, Wagner, Fletcher, & Gramzow, 1991). I submit that children begin to experience shame and guilt even earlier, as soon as they understand the significance of transgression against a standard and have a stable sense of self (Lewis, 1993a; see also Moskowitz, 1997). It may be important to differentiate between patterns of expression of shame and guilt even in early childhood, because the experience of and proneness to these emotions can lead to very different intra- and interpersonal consequences (Tangney, 1990, 1992).

Specifically, shamed individuals frequently become angry (Tangney et al., 1991; Tangney, 1995b), with self-reported maladaptive anger management strategies (Tangney, Wagner, et al., 1996; Tangney, 1995a). For instance, as the little girl and her teddy bear are forcefully extracted from the dirt, she feels rage at her parent for shaming her; she even kicks, bites, and squeals as she is dispatched to the tub. Shame-prone individuals also often lack empathy for others and blame others for the shame-inducing event (Tangney, 1991, 1995a, 1995b).

Hence, shame can motivate behaviors that interfere with interpersonal relationships. In fact, the tendency to feel shame about the entire self has been consistently linked to a range of psychological symptoms (Gramzow & Tangney, 1992; Tangney, Burggraf, & Wagner, 1995).

In contrast, guilt motivates corrective action rather than motivating avoidance:

> Three-year-old Erica, after clambering successfully to the top of the kitchen counter, turned to see her father's serious face. Knowing that climbing was a "big no," she quickly looked down, her whole body registering her guilt. She whispered, "I'm sorry, Daddy," and quietly but quickly climbed down.

Thus, in sharp contrast with shame, guilt is more likely to keep people constructively engaged in interpersonal situations. The tension and regret of guilt are more likely to lead to a desire to confess, apologize, and/or amend, even in very young children. This motivation for reparation derives from guilt's fairly persistent focus on the offending behavior and its harmful consequences to others.

During guilt, the self also remains relatively intact; it is unimpaired by shame-related global devaluations, and thus mobile to take reparative action. Children's and adults' "shame-free" guilt is linked to a range of more positive interpersonal dimensions, including other-oriented empathy, a tendency to accept responsibility for harming others, constructive responses to anger, and self-reported adherence to conventional standards of morality (Tangney, 1991, 1992, 1995a, 1995b; Tangney, Wagner, et al., 1996). This relatively clear picture of guilt's greater adaptiveness when compared to shame becomes murky when it fuses with shame or becomes so persistent that it immobilizes an individual (Tangney, 1996). It may also be true, but empirical evidence is needed, that personal styles of shame- or guilt-proneness do not become established until well into the grade-school-age range; work to determine the answer to this important question is progressing (Ferguson, 1996).

## Shame and Pride

Shame and pride do appear during the preschool period. Their prerequisites are in place. Lewis (1993a) asserts that the emotions of pride and shame require self-awareness, awareness of a rule that should be followed or will be broken (as in guilt), and a definite standard for one's own particular behavior. Thus the child evaluates his or her own behavior against this criterion: "*I* have done something dreadful or wonderful." This reference to a self-standard is central to the experience of shame or pride.

### Assessment of Shame and Pride

The actual measurement of shame and pride in young children has been difficult. There are no unique facial indicators necessary, so that investigators must rely heavily on behavior to infer the experience and expression for both emotions. Moreover, asking young children about their own experience of shame, guilt, or pride is complicated by their lack of verbal ability. The operational definitions that have been used are based on cultural consensus on body movement and posture, as well as verbalization.

Much of the early childhood research in the area has been conducted by Lewis and colleagues (e.g., Chen, Sullivan, & Lewis, 1995; Lewis, 1992; Lewis, Alessandri, & Sullivan, 1992) and by Stipek and colleagues (e.g., Stipek, Recchia, & McClintic, 1992). Both groups have presented young children with easy and difficult tasks, and have then observed the emotional responses of shame and pride that are implicit within success and failure experiences. For both research groups, shame is coded when the child's body seems "collapsed." In shame, the child's shoulders are hunched; hands are down and close to the body; and arms or hands are placed in front of the face or across the body. Also, shame is coded when a child shows avoidant postures with head and chin down, body to side or squirming, turning away, lowered eyes with gaze downward or askance, pouting, frowning, lower lip tucked between the teeth, withdrawal from the task situation, or negative verbal self-evaluations such as "I can't do it."[4]

> Erin wet on the bathroom floor because she waited too long to get to the bathroom. Her mother cried in exasperation, "Why did you wait so long? Now look what you've done!" Erin shrank down, turned partly away, and said softly, "I'm sorry, Mommy." She was experiencing shame.

Pride, conversely, is coded when the child adopts an open, erect posture, with shoulders back, head up, and/or arms open and up. Other behaviors indicating smiling, pointing at the outcome, applauding, verbalizing positive self-statements ("Look what I did!" "I did it!"), calling attention to the product, or looking up (presumably for confirmation).

> Later on the day of her "accident," Erin counted all the numbers in a book. Her mother exclaimed, "Very good! You knew every one of those!"

*Erin smiled, danced around, and read the numbers again. This time she felt proud.*

Hence, according to these definitions, both pride and shame have been observed as early as 27 months, and all children show these emotions by 42 months (see also Reissland & Harris, 1991). A recent breakthrough has occurred in asking children about their own experiences of shame (and guilt). Ferguson, Eyre, Stegge, Sorenson, and Everton (1997) have created a scenario-based measure, similar to that devised by Tangney (1990) for adults, which probes children's distinctive proneness shame, guilt, and ruminative guilt. Stories are presented to children as young as 5 years old, such as spilling juice on an aunt's rug. Children's predominant responses—in the case of the spilled juice, feeling bad, feeling so bad one can think of nothing else, or feeling dumb—map onto guilt, ruminative guilt, and shame, respectively. Although the measure is still in the development stage, its shame scale differentiates children with internalizing problems. Thus, it promises access to relatively young children's experience of social emotion.

### Moderators of the Experience of Pride and Shame

*Task Success and Failure.* Task success and failure conditions, as well as task difficulty, moderate the occurrence of shame and pride. The constellation of indicators for pride is shown most often after success, and is seen especially often after success on difficult tasks. Children show shame only after failure, not success, and especially after failure on easy tasks. Sadness and wariness do not differ across task conditions.

So expression of self-conscious emotions differs in conditions with differing implications for the self. In contrast, because their expression and experience are not intimately tied to a foundation of self-development, basic emotions such as sadness and fear are not expected to differ according to success or failure and task difficulty conditions. This empirical evidence strengthens the interpretation that shame and pride are unique, self-conscious emotions, not merely derivatives of the basic emotions (Chen et al., 1995). In sum, children show well-differentiated emotional and behavioral reactions to success and failure, quite early in the preschool period. The differences in these reactions suggest that specific contexts for pride and shame have been uncovered.

*Age and Internal Working Models.* Although researchers have uncovered very few age trends in preschoolers' expression of shame, Stipek et al. (1992) found that children under 42 months of age were more likely to look away from the experimenter when they failed, suggesting their concern with social evaluation and anticipation of a negative reaction. In contrast, the older children were twice as likely to pout or frown, consistent with "a more independent or internalized self-evaluation" (Stipek et al., 1992, p. 58). Thus, the experience of shame moves from being more externally to more internally based—more and more a "*self*-conscious" emotion.

This change in shame's experience over age should not be over-emphasized, however. In fact, the internal basis for shame may occur even earlier than Stipek and colleagues discerned. Malatesta et al.'s (1989) results suggest that shame or pride originates as early as 24 months of age. They assert that early expression of *positive* self-conscious emotion is associated with a stable concept of self and a sense of one's inherent worthiness, as captured in the internal working models of secure attachment relationships. For example, insecurely attached toddlers expressed more shame than securely attached toddlers while attributing negative emotions to photographs of other children and parents (Malatesta et al., 1989). Perhaps these toddlers internalized the negativity of their early parent–child interactions as follows: "I am not worthy of the care and positive regard of others; these people in the pictures probably think I am bad." Such an internal working model of self is certainly shame-promoting. Hence, Malatesta and colleagues reason, when insecure toddlers observe the negative emotions of the photographed children, their own very internally based shame is activated.

Stipek et al. (1992) offer an argument consistent with Malatesta et al.'s notion that shame originates from internal conceptions about relationships with others. They reason that toddlers and preschoolers will rarely have experienced direct criticism for failing at developmental tasks such as putting a puzzle together or embedding plastic cups (this may not be true for all children!), but that even very young children want to please grownups. These youngsters experience failure and associated shame not only when the self is threatened, but also when they are not following rules or living up to adults' expectations. Although this assertion does ground the young child's experience of shame within relationships, as in Malatesta and colleagues' work, it also again obfuscates the differentiation between shame and guilt. Presumably, simply not following rules would result in guilt—not the shame-like patterns evidenced after failure by so many of the participants in Stipek et al.'s studies—unless breaking an adult's rule was seen as *failing in the relationship*.

In short, age-related changes in the bases for shame are as yet only tantalizing. Perhaps the arguments of Malatesta et al. and Stipek et al. can be integrated by asserting that shame is experienced when a child with a shame-based internal working model of self fails another person or does not follow rules. Similar to the internal working models of others postulated by attachment theory, this internalization could happen fairly early. The experience of shame could be more dependent on the response of adults earlier in the preschool period, but relatively stable and independent of adults' reactions later. More effort should be expended to examine these viewpoints empirically, and to define more clearly the roles of age and internal working models of self in the experience and expression of shame and pride.

*Gender.* Gender differences in the expression of shame, pride, and guilt also emerge early. Preschool girls show more shame than boys do (Lewis et al., 1992; Stipek et al., 1992); they are more likely than boys to frown after failure. There are also gender differences in pride, with girls showing more positive expressions after success (Stipek et al., 1992). Moreover, the pattern of associations among self-conscious emotions differs for boys and girls. In Lewis et al.'s (1992) study, guilt- and shame-proneness were related for girls; if a girl expressed one of these negative self-conscious emotions, she was also likely to exhibit the other. Boys' self-conscious emotions did not show this pattern of association; their expression of guilt was unrelated to evidence of their shame. Instead, shame-prone boys were *less* likely to show pride, as if their bad feelings about themselves precluded their good feelings of pride.

*Summary*

Adults want to remedy the negative social relationships that inspire shame in young children, to avoid any difficult outcomes associated with shame, and to foster the positive self-experiences that engender pride. Clearly, much more effort is needed to delineate precisely how these emotions are expressed. Researchers need to vigorously investigate the possibility of shame-proneness, and the correlates of shame, in children this young. How does the frequent experience of shame affect social transactions with peers?

# Guilt

Young children are impulsive, sometimes do not comply with rules, and are often not competent enough to succeed at certain tasks. So they experience (and express) guilt or shame, or at least similar rudimentary emotions.

*A mother describes an incident of her preschool son's guilt: "James [aged 4] hit his 5-year-old cousin. In a firm and probably angry voice, I told him, 'We don't use our hands to hurt.' He said, 'I'm sorry, it was an accident.' He then sat on the stairs alone for a couple of minutes, and got up and apologized."*

Hoffman (1984) suggests that empathy is motivated by feeling responsible for, or guilty about, another's plight. In this view, interpersonal guilt results from the simultaneous feeling of sympathy toward another's distress, and the awareness of being the cause of that distress—such as realizing that one's misbehavior dismays one's parent (Zahn-Waxler & Radke-Yarrow, 1990). Whether empathy is a precondition for guilt, whether guilt is a precondition for empathy, or whether both arise together is a matter of some debate.

## Assessment of Guilt

In any case, evidence of guilt appears during the second year of life (Hoffman, 1984). But, as with shame, the study of guilt in young children has been a challenge. Cole, Barrett, and Zahn-Waxler (1992; see also Barrett, Zahn-Waxler, & Cole, 1993) have created ingenious quasi-naturalistic paradigms; for example, a doll breaks and a cup of juice spills, ostensibly through the fault of the child. While experiencing these mishaps, 2-year-olds show more negative emotion than during free play, and often attempt to make reparations. The authors take this pattern of responses as evidence of guilt.

Narrative story methods have also been used to elucidate young children's experience of guilt. In these methods, children use dioramas and dolls to complete stories about fighting with one's sibling over a bicycle, an angry mother, a crying baby, and their mother's crying. They express their own experience of guilt in the themes they enact. These themes, including negative emotion, self-blame, and desire for reparation, become more frequent with age (Zahn-Waxler, Kochanska, Krupnick, & McKnew, 1990). Children act out feeling bad and responsible about these actions, and seeking to make amends. When the mother doll is crying, a girl may have the child doll give the mother doll a kiss and say, "Mommy, I am sorry, I didn't mean to hurt your feelings."

## Summary

Again, more effort is needed to delineate the specific patterns of expressing this complex emotion. Investigations of the possibility of guilt-proneness, and of the moderators and correlates of guilt in children this young, are also needed. If guilt has a powerful association with reparations and prosocial behavior, then it is incumbent upon adults to assist children in its experience and successful resolution.

Similarly, potentially deleterious effects of persistent or shame-fused guilt need to be specified.

## Embarrassment

Although embarrassment, like shame, appears early in life, it differs from shame. As with shame and pride, researchers link the emergence of embarrassment to requisite self-knowledge; unlike either of these self-conscious emotions, embarrassment is also affected by the quality of an audience's behavior. That is, children are unlikely to be embarrassed before they have a sense of self, but in order to experience embarrassment, they must also perceive that an audience (either real or imagined) would make fun of their actions.

### Assessment of Embarrassment

Very little was known until recently about the differentiation of embarrassment from the other self-conscious emotions, especially shame. Lewis and his colleagues have begun to delve into the short-term developmental course of and necessary conditions for toddlers' embarrassment. In two investigations, four embarrassment-eliciting situations were assessed: viewing oneself in a mirror, being praised overmuch, and being invited to dance with one's mother or an experimenter (Lewis, Stanger, Sullivan, & Barone, 1991; Lewis, Sullivan, Stanger, & Weiss, 1989). Clearly, each eliciting situation contained elements of self-consciousness and the possibility of an audience that might ridicule a child.

Embarrassment was indexed by silly smiles, giggling, hand gestures, and body movements—especially by smiling while averting one's gaze or touching one's hair, clothing, or face. This emotion was more evident in the four situations of self-exposure noted above than in any other experimental situations, and was more often seen in older toddlers and in children who recognized themselves in the mirror. Thus, such self-referential ability is necessary, but not sufficient, for the expression of embarrassment.

### Audience Behavior: A Moderator the Experience of Embarrassment

Another important element of young children's experience of embarrassment is the presence of an audience that is likely to poke fun at one's shortcomings (Bennett, 1989). Such an audience, and especially a derisive one, will elicit this emotion. Bennett asked children to report how they would react in situations involving either a rule violation or a solo performance. The situations included either no audience, a passive audience, or a derisive audience. Children aged 5 to 8 years said that they would be unlikely to be embarrassed in the presence of a passive audience, but they felt quite differently about the ridiculing audience. Hence, imagining actual reactions of the other persons is important to young children; in this emotional reasoning, as in their understanding of the physical world, they are quite concrete.

To experience embarrassment, children need an actual derisive audience, rather than mere self-ridicule. Preschoolers' embarrassment can stem from the actual *punitive behavior* of the deriding audience, rather than from negative *self*-evaluations emanating from the derision. In a second study (Bennett & Gillingham, 1991), children were again asked how they would feel after rule violation and solo performance, but a supportive audience was pitted against a deriding one. Five-year-olds focused on the supportive or punitive quality of the audience's behavior, rather than on the self-evaluations that the audience could engender; they more often cited embarrassment in the deriding audience condition. Although it is a painfully experienced self-conscious emotion, embarrassment differs from shame in that others' negative evaluations are more important than one's own.

### Summary

External, rather than internal, psychological grounds are invoked as causing preschoolers' experiences of embarrassment. To complicate this picture slightly, Lewis continues to underscore the inclusion of embarrassment's requisite self-knowledge, as in "I know the punitive, deriding audience is laughing at *me*" (Lewis, 1992; Lewis et al., 1992). As with shame, then, the experience of embarrassment becomes more and more internal with time; even young children can experience embarrassment when they *imagine* a deriding audience. And, as with the other social and self-conscious emotions, more investigations are warranted of how embarrassment relates to other patterns of expressiveness and to social competence. Are easily embarrassed children more prone to the even more pernicious experience of shame? Does the experience of embarrassment put young children at risk of negotiating social interactions poorly?

## A CAUTION REGARDING SELF-CONSCIOUS AND SOCIAL EMOTIONS

These expressive developments are most intriguing; they demonstrate the potential sophistication of young children's emotional experience. A caveat is in order here, however. Reconsider the argument of whether young children really *experience* emotions as adults do—especially those emotions requiring a concept of self, a set of standards as a point of comparison, the ability to distinguish self and behavior, and life experience (Tangney, 1998). As Tangney asserts, these emotions are about the self (and others). Important cognitive milestones continue to be intrinsic aspects of empathy, shame, guilt, pride, and embarrassment. These milestones "emerge in childhood, first as a glimmer of an ability, and later . . . as increasingly complex and elaborated capacities that almost certainly transform our experience of the emotions to which they are intimately linked" (Tangney, 1998, p. 10).

So conceptual and methodological problems still exist in the study of social and self-conscious emotions. Merely applying an emotion label to the behavior of a 3-year-old, such as the label "shame," does not mean that the 3-year-old experiences the emotion state of shame the way adults do. To return to an earlier example, Leah *may* feel ashamed when forced to recite her rhyme, or at least may exhibit shame-related behaviors, such as looking at the floor. Even though there is a similarity in the essence of her and her father's experiences—the core of affective continuity—her experience is probably not the same "shame" that her father feel when he fails as a professor. Much more thinking is necessary about how to access the emotional experience of young children, so that developmentalists do not fall into a trap of forgetting that important phenomena both *stay the same* and *change* as children develop. Adults' zeal at identifying these kernels of affective continuity should not discourage efforts to provide a truer picture of the changes inherent in the development of these intricate emotions.

## VOLUNTARY MANAGEMENT OF EMOTIONAL EXPRESSION

Voluntary management of facial expressions also emerges during the preschool period (Field & Walden, 1982; Malatesta et al., 1989; Lewis, Sullivan, & Vasen, 1987). Children's first attempts at intentionally and successfully posing facial expressions often occur when a rule of self-display or social display, or deceiving others about one's "true" feelings, is necessary. A social display rule functions when a 5-year-old boy, given a tiny portion of meatloaf, smiles rather than yelling at Grandma that he wants more. To protect herself and avoid punishment, a 4-year-old girl may behave according to a self-display rule, feigning an unconcerned expression when she is discovered atop the kitchen counter (unlike Erica in an earlier example).

Importantly, some of these new skills in voluntary control of facial expressions serve the function of *maintaining* rather than *derailing* social interactions. Children also learn when to display emotions that facilitate social interaction. Such voluntary management of expressiveness is important because it aids even very young children in their coping efforts. Control of facial expression is a vital contributor to social competence, then, through the ability to manage the nuances of emotion-laden interactions. With these intentional abilities, the child feels better and more in control, and is also more able to enact appropriate social interaction.

## Posed Expressions

One of the first manifestations of voluntary expressive control is children's ability to pose specific emotional expressions, whether at an adult's request or during play. Thus, preschoolers can also pose emotional expressions:

> *Manuel displays very contrived anger while pretending to be a police officer with Bobby and Andrea: "Move it, buster." They seem to know he is just feigning anger and simply ignore him.*

This voluntary modulation and control of expression through posing form a foundation for the modification of emotional expressiveness in the service of display rules or deception (Lewis, 1993a, 1993b).

Young children have sufficient voluntary control of their emotional expressiveness to pose specific expressions, but this ability does change over the toddler-through-preschool age range. In research by Lewis's group, 2- through 5-year-olds, as well as adults, were asked to pose happiness, sadness, anger, fear, surprise, and disgust (Lewis, 1993b; Lewis et al., 1987). Two-year-olds did not accurately pose any of the expressions. Three-year-olds, termed a transitional age group, posed happiness and surprise; the accuracy of posing happiness did not increase after this age (see also Field & Walden, 1982). More improvement occurred between 3 and 4 years. The 4- and 5-year-olds were less skilled than adults only in producing surprise and anger expressions. No age group, including adults, was able to pose fear or disgust well according to discrete emotion criteria, but preschoolers tended to err by making a "scary" rather than a "scared" face.

Videotaped posed expressions were grouped into complete expressions, which included all components of the target expression, and partial expressions, which included only some of the components of the target expressions. Partial poses were consistently more frequent than complete poses for sadness, fear, and disgust, across ages. Why are negative expressions so consistently difficult to demonstrate at will (see also Field & Walden, 1982)? One plausible explanation is that negative expressiveness requires more control of facial muscles. Yet another credible interpretation is that children have deficiencies in differentiating how negative expressions look or are made (Cole, 1985; Denham & Couchoud, 1990b). A third explanation for these developmental patterns is that children are already exposed to socialization pressures to suppress negative expressiveness. Perhaps preschoolers are showing us their capabilities to both to suppress and to dissemble expressiveness when they demonstrate difficulty posing negative expressions in these investigations. Even when asked, they may be reluctant to generate or even to acknowledge expressions of sadness and anger; some flatly state, "But I'm not mad," or "I don't want to be sad" (Cole, 1985).

Although these spontaneous verbalizations hint at a socialization hypothesis, rather than the hypotheses of emotion knowledge or facial muscle control, this link is not irrefutable. The children's comments also highlight their efforts to avoid the uncomfortable felt experience that is for them still inextricable from their expressiveness. In support of this argument, even emotionally knowledgeable and motorically skilled adults have more trouble simulating negative expressiveness. In any case, young children's growing ability to pose expressive patterns can be taken as evidence of their increasing voluntary control of their own expressiveness.

## Control of Expressiveness and Adherence to Display Rules

As voluntary management of emotional expressiveness expands, display rules come to be employed. Children learn to use affective displays strategically—to substitute, mask, minimize, or maximize patterns of expressiveness according to cultural expectations and for self-preservative purposes (Ekman & Friesen, 1975). All of these abilities involve knowledge of when, where, and how to control the display of emotions. Children may first minimize or maximize expressive patterns that are already within their repertoire. The mastery of substitution or masking strategies is achieved later, because more cognitive ability and facial muscle control are required to change the expression of emotion from that which is experienced (Saarni & von Salisch, 1993).

A surge in both understanding and utilization of display strategies takes place during the elementary school years. Three possible reasons exist for whatever difficulties preschoolers do have in using display rules. First, although they learn *verbal* strategies to discount emotions early, young children obtain less feedback on how to modify *facial* and *vocal* displays. They can learn facial and vocal display rules more readily through observation of others and through indirect feedback. Second, they need to learn how to inhibit both facial muscle movement and vocalization in order to adhere to display rules. Third, preschoolers also experience relative difficulty in making critical self-evaluations (e.g., "I need to change my angry display here for Grandma's sake"). Complete acquisition of the skills inherent in all these factors take time.

So, until recently, there has been far more research into grade school children's display rule usage than into preschoolers'. Nonetheless, preschoolers' usage of both self-protective and other-oriented display rules is more sophisticated than previously assumed. Use of naturalistic rather than laboratory contexts allows researchers to witness preschoolers' true abilities in this area.

Because of this need for more ecologically valid investigations, researchers are utilizing ingenious paradigms to identify how very young children use display rules. In studies using these new methods, evidence appears very early for expressiveness patterns' fit with cultural display and self-display rules. Toddlers already exhibit expressive patterns that signal dampening of negative emotions, such as wrinkled brow, compressed lips, and lip biting (Malatesta et al., 1989). They are minimizing emotions that could potentially cause problems for themselves and others. From this very young age onward children also maximize expressions that serve to dramatize distress to get assistance, such as the anger exhibited during a sibling conflict (Dunn, Bretherton, & Munn, 1987), or to dominate by their rage shown on the playground (Blurton-Jones, 1967). They are modifying the expression of their emotions to serve specific goals.

## Functions of Display Rule Usage

Maximization serves the self-protective function of enlisting aid and/or gaining adults' attention and compliance with their wishes. For instance, a 3-year-old girl may begin to cry loudly several moments *after* she bumps her elbow on the lunch table—that is, when her day care teacher reenters the room. Toddlers also use substituted or masked expressions strategically for the self-serving functions of joking and teasing (Dunn et al., 1987; Dunn & Munn, 1985; Lewis, 1993b). For example, after a 4-year-old boy holds his sister's blanket in his hand and feigns a sad look, he may begin to laugh at his own mockery.

Display rules are also used by preschoolers to smooth "bumpy" social interactions with peers and adults. Knowing when to minimize anger by showing only furrowed brows or pursed lips could help avoid a fight. There are empirical data that the upper facial muscles' "social" smile increases in frequency across the 2- to 4-year-old age period, but only when the child is interacting with same-sex peers (Cheyne, 1976). Presumably this smile is voluntarily controlled in order to initiate contact and optimize the fun of shared activity.

Display rules are also used in the service of kindness by preschool-age siblings (Reissland & Harris, 1991). Five-year-olds mask their pride more often than their 3-year-old younger brothers and sisters do during competitive game-playing interactions. Presumably they do not want to make their younger siblings feel inept, or to "rub it in" when they win.

## Moderators of Display Rule Usage: Context and Gender

But all this maximization and minimization and masking are complicated. How does the young child come to *when* to enact *which* pattern of voluntary expression management? There must be some guides along the way! Two such guides could be (1) the cultural rules of context, and (2) the gender of oneself and others in an interaction.

As children develop, the identities of their partners in interaction become increasingly important for the use of display rules (Zeaman & Garber, 1996). First-graders endorse more emotional control around peers than around parents or when alone. Peers often reject, ridicule, or reprimand a friend who shows sadness, anger, or pain. Thus, there is probably a complex association between children's understanding of emotions and display rule usage. As children age, they become better at reasoning about the antecedents and consequences of, for example, crying in front of a friend. They also come to distinguish the emotional experience of themselves and others; for instance, they feel scared while they cry, but their friends feel amused. Finally, they better implement their emotion knowledge, when appropriate, in the service of display rules (Fuchs & Thelen, 1988). Preschoolers are just beginning to discern these understandings.

So young children may be controlling the expression of emotion, but not necessarily its experience, to conform with their culture's "feeling rules." They probably also conform to gender stereotype expectations for emotional expressiveness and its control. To examine this possibility, preschoolers were given a disappointing toy as a gift, and their ensuing facial expressions were microanalytically coded (Cole, 1986). Girls were already spontaneously controlling the outward expression of emotion; boys showed the only sad expressions, whereas girls showed more positive and neutral displays. But when the experimenter queried the children about how they felt about the gift and their willingness to trade it for something better, most children—both boys and girls—reported actually feeling sad or mad. They said that they would be happy to trade the disappointing gift for a more attractive one. The experience and expression of emotions were differentiated by girls only.

In a second study, only girls participated; the examiner remained in the room with some of them after giving the unattractive gift, but for others she left (Cole, 1986). Girls smiled more when the examiner remained, suggesting that the function of such smiling is indeed to conform to expectations of "appropriate" social behavior by masking a negative emotion in the service of politeness. Again, these girls may have modified their expressiveness to conform more closely to a standard of socially appropriate behavior.

But usage of display rules is flexibly context-sensitive. In one situation, display rules may pressure children to show socially appropriate expressions despite emotional experience ("Don't show what you feel; show what you don't feel"). In another, display rules may allow and encourage children to show what they experience in order to obtain support. In neither case are display rules necessary when children are alone, because no one is receiving the managed emotional signal. Which sort of display rule is invoked when someone *is* around depends on who that someone is.

Making these contextual distinctions is a tall order. These complexities also depend on gender. When children were asked how they would control emotional expressiveness around parents or peers or when alone, first-grade girls were much *more* likely to say that they would show their sadness and pain (Zeaman & Garber, 1996). They were more apt than their male counterparts to see other people as understanding and accepting of these feelings.

Thus, girls see the demonstration of distress as appropriate in order to get support, whereas boys focus on perceived negative reactions of others. Similarly, girls consider the discomfort of another person in the gift paradigm, and boys seem not to. Boys' use, or nonuse, of display rules is differentiated along different dimensions than girls'. Caring adults need to be conscious of how boys and girls differ in their perceptions of the acceptability of certain expressive patterns, and in their notions of how others react to these displays.

## Deception, or Self-Protective Expressiveness

The foregoing examples of display rule usage highlight the strategic control of emotional expressiveness in order to attain a personal goal, render a dyadic interaction more successful, or minimize another person's discomfort. *Deceptive* masking of expressiveness also takes place within the preschool period. Such deception serves the function of avoiding guilt, shame, and possible punishment (Lewis, Stanger, &

Sullivan, 1989). In Lewis and colleagues' studies, children watched an experimenter set up an elaborate toy. They were told that they were going to be allowed to look at it and play with it later, but that they were *not* to look at it while the experimenter left to do some work. Each child was given nothing else to do during this period. Five minutes later, the experimenter returned, stared pointedly at the child, and asked, "Did you peek?" The children's actual behavior with the toy, as well as their facial and behavioral responses to the experimenter's question, were coded.

In reality, only 10% of the children complied with the experimenter's instructions not to look at the attractive toy—but of those who did peek, two-thirds either lied about doing so or did not respond to the question. It is vital to note that coding of the videotaped facial expression of deniers and nondeniers did *not* differ. No one showed guilt—and deception really did occur. At the moment of questioning about peeking, the deceptive children did not show any expressive differences from those who told the truth. Facial expressive elements such as relaxed face, smiling, frowning, nervous touching, biting of the lips, and gaze aversion did not distinguish deniers from nondeniers. Moreover, judges could not reliably identify deniers versus nondeniers, regardless of the age or gender of a child, or the age, gender, and experience of a judge.

There were many children who were deceptive, but again there was a sex difference in those who chose to mask their guilt and fear: Girls followed the experimenter's orders much more often than boys, but boys were far more likely than girls to admit their transgression. Hence, girls formed the vast majority of deniers and nonresponders— that is, deceivers. Lewis and colleagues' and Cole's findings are convergent therefore: Young girls precociously use both display rules and dissemblance.

Hence, preschoolers, mostly girls, can effectively mask expressions of apprehension about the discovery of their transgressions. Lewis suggests that the function of this dissemblance is self-preservative, masking fear of punishment and guilt over disobeying.

## Summary

Conformity to display rules clearly surfaces during the preschool period (see also Cole, Zahn-Waxler, & Smith, 1994). There is evidence of maximization, minimization, and masking, following the proscriptions and prescriptions of children's cultures, and also self-serving goals. However, as Cole (1985) asserts, findings suggest that most "*nonconscious* adjustments [in expressive patterns] implying tacit personal and/or cultural display rules. The preschooler's cognitive limitations in self-reflective, inferential, and abstract social reasoning may render such tacit knowledge inaccessible" (p. 285; emphasis added).

At the same time, it is important to underscore that young children are beginning to comprehend that emotional displays may be modified; more will be said on this topic in Chapter 3. They also evidence some specific strategies to do so, especially in naturalistic investigations. Because of the potential importance of maximization, minimization, masking, and substitution of emotions to social competence (or its lack), much more research is needed to flesh out the intriguing results of the studies reported here. Nevertheless, adults should be aware of young children's potential for display rule usage and deception, if discerning their charges' true feelings is necessary.

## CHAPTER SUMMARY

Much change in emotional expressiveness occurs during the toddler-to-preschool period. Personal styles of emotional expressiveness become established, and children gain flexibility in using their expression of basic emotions strategically (e.g., using vocal and facial channels differentially). Moreover, self-conscious and social emotions such as empathy, guilt, shame, and embarrassment appear. Voluntary management of emotions also increases, as evidenced through the posing of expressions, the following of cultural pre- and proscriptions about expressive patterns, and personal dissemblance.

In short, children entering kindergarten are becoming masterful in expressing emotions as goal-directed behaviors and as social signals.

> Byron's mixture of disgust, goofy happiness, and a tinge of anger gets his message across: "I think you are weird to reject me from your play, guys. I am unfazed–but don't cross me in the future." Sandra's exaggerated fear expression while her teacher reads a scary story conveys a different message; it invites other kindergartners to join her in the delicious experience of "courting" fear in a safe environment.

These changes hold implications for parents and teachers alike. Children of early grade school age are often much more difficult to "read" than preschoolers, because some of their emotions are masked, dissembled, or blended. More effort is required to know what these older children are experiencing emotionally. Their emotional lives are also more complex, with guilt, shame, and embarrassment requiring careful attention from the adults in their lives.

## NOTES

1. It certainly is difficult to access the emotional experience of young children accurately. I have trouble imagining asking a preschooler, "What are you feeling right now?", and getting much more than a bald answer of "Bad," "Good," "Sad," or "I don't know." Even this limited information is useful, of course, but verbal and cognitive capacities seem to place severe restrictions on preschoolers' production of well-differentiated self-reports of emotion. A few researchers have moved toward potential success in this area, however, and some parents can sensitively determine their children's "real" feelings. Fabes and Eisenberg (1992) have interviewed young children *in vivo* about the causes of their anger. Dunn and Hughes (1998) have interviewed preschoolers about what causes their own emotions, as well as those of their mothers, siblings, and friends (see also Denham & Zoller, 1991). Of course, during these interviews the children are *remembering* emotions, not *experiencing* them. Nonetheless, they are at least able to consider their own emotional experience, and therein lies the possibility of somehow creating imaginative, ecologically valid ways of discussing current feelings with preschoolers. Alternatively, viewing videotapes and reliving affect could be one way of validating a preschooler's emotional experience after the fact. Similarly, although physiological means are not yet sophisticated enough to identify discrete emotions, there is promise in the approach of marrying convergent measurements of physiology and self-report. Developmentalists need continued support in this difficult endeavor.

2. Of course, as children learn to pose expressions of emotions voluntarily (a topic I turn to later in this chapter), it is possible for them to "use" emotions to get their way in interactions with adults. The point here is that adults should at least reflect on the multiple adaptive functions possible for any emotion they observe, and use this information to guide their own responses.

3. In espousing this functionalist view, I do not dismiss the bioevolutionary origin of emotional expressiveness; nor do I overlook the biological bases of emotional expressiveness. But my background as an applied developmental psychologist drives me to look for practical ways of understanding phenomena of development. At this point we cannot change a child's inheritance, or in many cases change his or her physiology. In contrast, the functional viewpoint, with its emphasis on events in the child's life and on the child's goals and action tendencies, bolsters our understanding of toddlers' and preschoolers' lives in relation to others.

4. Others would include indicators such as covering the eyes, mouth, or face, and touching of various parts of the face (Tesman, Shepard, & VanValkenburgh, 1993).

## Chapter 3

# Understanding of Emotions

$P$reschoolers can show knowledge of the causes and consequences of common emotions:

> *Rosie is playing with a girl doll, who is in her bed in the dollhouse. She
> speaks for the doll: "I'm having a bad dream! A big tiger is chasing me!
> Mommy! Mommy!" Rosie quickly whisks the mother doll into the room.
> "Wake up, sweetie, wake up! There's no more, there's no tigers chasing
> you."*
>     *Rosie then brings the mother and daughter dolls into the dollhouse
> kitchen. The girl doll says, "Thank you, Mommy. I want to get you new
> high-heeled shoes to make you happy!"*

As noted in Chapter 2, toddlers and preschoolers express emotions
vividly and frequently. Their own and others' emotions are central
experiences in their lives. So the unfolding of sophisticated emotion
understanding is quite critical for young children. First and foremost,
this understanding supports preschoolers' attempts to deal with and
communicate about the emotions they experience. Despite his generally limited use of words, a 3-year-old boy can speak with great intensity
about his sadness when he lost his favorite stuffed cat: " 'Wow' gone.
I cried."
    Second, particularly because of their verbal limitations, emotions

are extraordinarily important social signals for young children. Emotions are immediate, salient, and important in their social transactions. Thus, as their cognitive and language abilities mature, preschoolers almost unwittingly construct coherent understandings about their own and others' feelings (Bretherton & Beeghly, 1982; Bretherton, Fritz, Zahn-Waxler, & Ridgeway, 1986; Harris, 1989, 1993). Young children learn the facial expressions, vocal patterns, goals, and likely behaviors associated with a variety of emotions (Campos & Barrett, 1984). They work out the meaning of emotions by focusing on the relation between desire and reality: "Sadness is when I want something but can't have it, like when Mommy says I can't have pie" (Denham & Zoller, 1991). Even 2-year-olds begin to understand that wanting and getting lead to happiness, whereas wanting and not getting lead to sadness (Harris, Johnson, Hutton, Andrews, & Cooke, 1989; Wellman & Woolley, 1990; Yuill, 1984). Children of this age also come to know that the anger felt by themselves and others often involves being in an undesired state, along with a gruff vocal tone, lowered brows, and a tendency to attack physically or verbally. An understanding of anger allows young children to interpret high-level anger in others as a signal to "get out of the way" (Denham, 1986).

Researchers have increasingly probed more deeply into young children's conceptions about emotions (e.g., Denham, 1986; Fabes, Eisenberg, McCormick, & Wilson, 1988; Strayer, 1986). Findings reveal that changes in emotion understanding occur from toddlerhood through the preschool years. These changes are evident in nine areas of children's emotion understanding, which I will describe in turn:

- Labeling emotional expressions, both verbally and nonverbally.
- Identifying emotion-eliciting situations.
- Inferring the causes of emotion-eliciting situations, as well as the consequences of specific emotional responses.
- Using emotion language to describe their own emotional experiences and to clarify those of others.
- Recognizing that others' emotional experience can differ from their own.
- Becoming aware of emotion regulation strategies.
- Beginning to develop a knowledge of emotion display rules.
- Beginning to develop a knowledge of how more than one emotion may be felt simultaneously, even when these emotions conflict or are ambivalent.
- Beginning to understand complex social and self-conscious emotions (e.g., guilt).

## LABELING EMOTIONAL EXPRESSIONS

To show that they understand emotions and the cultural scripts associated with them, children must first distinguish among and name the common expressions associated with emotional experience. Preschoolers are already fairly adept at labeling emotional expressions, and become increasingly able over the period. Knowledge of basic emotional expressions is solid by the end of the preschool period, whether evaluated by expressions that are presented pictorially (e.g., Camras & Allison, 1985; Denham & Couchoud, 1990b), in photographs (Field & Walden, 1982), or "live" (Felleman, Barden, Carlson, Rosenberg, & Masters, 1983).

Specifically, preschoolers' abilities to verbally label and nonverbally recognize emotional expressions increase from 2 to $4\frac{1}{2}$ years of age (Denham & Couchoud, 1990b). In one study, we developed a contextually valid measure that involved puppets, both to capture children's attention and to embed a realistic situation within ongoing social interaction. Children were first shown four flannel faces on which prototypical emotion expressions of happiness, sadness, anger, and fear were drawn. Our findings with this methodology revealed that 2- through 5-year-olds pointed to or named emotional expressions. However, older children identified emotional expressions more accurately than younger ones, and for both groups receptive identification exceeded expressive identification. In addition, recognition of happy expressions was greater than recognition of negative emotions, and labeling of happy and sad expressions exceeded labeling of either anger or fear. Other researchers report a similar progression in preschoolers' identification of happy, sad, and angry faces, voices, and faces with voices (Camras & Allison, 1985; Stifter & Fox, 1987).

An interesting finding was noted by Camras and Allison (1985). In their study of preschoolers' understanding of emotional expressions, verbal identification was better than nonverbal for both fear and disgust. This finding reverses the usual trend for receptive and expressive understanding. Perhaps children see very little visual evidence of fear and disgust in their environments, but have been taught about them verbally.

Emotional situations and attendant facial expressions may be learned together. The first distinction learned may be the one between being happy and not happy, or feeling good versus bad or sad (Bullock & Russell, 1984, 1985, 1986). An understanding of anger and fear then emerges from the not happy/sad category. My research suggests that preschoolers often confuse negative emotions; Bullock and Russell, too, find "fuzzy borders" for negative emotion concepts. Young children's initial categories of emotion are also broader than those of adults'. This is so even though children and adults usually share similar sets of central defining characteristics for each basic emotion. What differs is that young children's categories include more peripheral concepts.

One foundation for the progression in understanding happy versus not happy/angry/fearful expressions is a perceptual one that involves the salience of the mouth (Cunningham & Odom, 1986). Kindergartners were shown facial photographs of an unfamiliar adult expressing anger, disgust, fear, joy, and shame. Recall of the photos was cued by probe photographs that varied in presentation of mouth, eyes, or nose. Children remembered expressive information from the mouth region first, eye region second, and nose region last. The happy–not happy distinction was identified by mouth expressions, which were the most salient feature isolated in this study. Eye region differences, the next most salient, differentiated among sadness, anger, and fear. It is reasonable that young children first differentiate an emotion whose prominent feature is the mouth—happiness. This initial learning is followed by emotional expressions for the negative emotions, which differ with respect to the eye region. The progression of comprehending happy expressions first and gradually teasing apart the various negative expressions is well substantiated.

As young children become increasingly able to discern important differences among expressions of emotions, the differentiation becomes a vital component of their overall understanding of emotions. Comprehension of emotional expressions can be seen as the perceptual bedrock for further understanding of emotions. As such, it stands preschoolers in good stead, giving them an initial ability to think and talk about emotional issues, including their eliciting situations.

## IDENTIFYING EMOTION-ELICITING SITUATIONS

Emotional expressions and their elicitors are inextricably intertwined, and both are vital components of emotional experience (Lewis & Michalson, 1983). To be able to comprehend their own or others' emotions, children must become familiar with and recognize the common eliciting situations for basic emotions. Overall, understanding of causal factors in emotional situations improves over the preschool period. As with the identification of expressions, happy and sad situations are easiest for children to interpret, whereas incorrect responses, such as "sad" or "don't know" errors, occur often for other negative emotions (Denham & Couchoud, 1990b; Fabes et al., 1991).

In general, a developmental progression similar to that for perceiving and labeling emotional expressions exists for comprehending the common situations for basic emotions. Young children first differentiate situations they call "happy" from those they call "not happy" or "sad," then begin to distinguish "angry" situations. In my studies, children eagerly and easily fasten the happy face on the puppet who is receiving ice cream or going to the zoo. Clearly, these acts mirror their own delight in experiencing these situations. Interestingly, many children at first tend to use the sad face for all the negative situations—being left by a sibling who wants to play with someone else, having to eat a disliked food, or having a block construction destroyed. Little by little, however, children clearly separate angry situations from sad ones.

Fear expressions present preschool children with the most difficulty in both accurate identification and situation comprehension (Brody & Harrison, 1987). Difficulty in understanding fear elicitors has many causes. Reasons include the complex brow/eye/mouth movements in the facial expression of fear, the infrequency of children's exposure to peak fear expressions, and the idiosyncratic views preschoolers have of fear's causes (Denham & Zoller, 1991; Strayer, 1986). Young children talk eloquently about such causes of fear as monsters, witches, darkness, and masks (Lieberman, 1993). In contrast, they refer far less frequently to more common, reality-based fear-producing experiences, such as falling while learning to ride a bicycle. They often include these situations with sadness-inducing ones, suggesting that they know fear-eliciting events are negative; however, they seem unable or unwilling to acknowledge the potential harm involved.

Thus, young children understand more and more about the common eliciting situations for basic emotions—a vital component of their overall understanding. The trend of comprehending happy situations followed by sad, angry, and fearful situations is clear. Understanding these basic emotions is particularly adaptive for preschoolers, because they witness and experience fairly vivid, clear demonstrations of these very feelings (see Chapter 2). Indeed, a preschool boy may experience many emotions in a day—great joy when his best friend brings in his puppy for "show and tell"; sadness when another peer tells him, "You can't play"; and, finally, anger when his mother comes to take him home before he is ready. But young children go even further than recognizing the expressions and eliciting situations for basic emotions. They make more complex attributions about emotions' causes, and reason more intricately about their consequences for behavior.

## COMPREHENDING CAUSES AND CONSEQUENCES OF EMOTIONS

Young children begin to use the contextual information found in their everyday experiences to figure out why happiness, sadness, and anger occur. They build upon their early understanding of basic emotional situations to create more intricate scenarios depicting specific persons' particular feelings (Dunn & Hughes, 1998). The causes they cite for the most familiar emotions are often similar to ones given by adults (Strayer, 1986; Fabes et al., 1991). Their explanations are particularly accurate when interpersonal and environmental event themes are involved: "Getting hit makes me angry," "Going to the playground makes me happy." Young children also realize the consequences of an emotion; for instance, a securely attached 3-year-old girl knows that a parent will comfort her when she is upset. Clearly, knowing why an emotion is expressed and what its aftermath is likely to be aids a child in learning to regulate the behavior and affect of self and others. I now detail these important abilities, with particular emphasis on understanding the emotions of self, peers, and family.

### Comprehending Causes of Specific Emotions

Preschoolers' understanding of the causes of emotion is impressive, particularly when their knowledge is compared with that of toddlers. They form reasonably coherent, internally consistent categories of emotion–situation linkages describing the lives of themselves, peers, and parents. Although these linkages often correspond at least broadly to the causal understandings of older children and adults, there are distinct differences. Young preschoolers' notions about the causes of emotions frequently do not specifically match those of adults. Three-year-olds, but not 4- and 5-year-olds, often give idiosyncratic reasons for emotions, such as "I was sad when we had a snack," "I was scared about a lost baby in the forest," or "I was angry because I get angry" (Denham & Zoller, 1991; Fabes et al., 1991; Strayer, 1986). Some of these idiosyncratic reasons make good sense phenomenologically when the situation is analyzed in detail. For instance, the child who claimed she was sad when a snack was served at day care had actually disliked the day's offering.

Clearly, even young children have an ample foundation of knowledge in this area. This budding awareness of the individuality of emotion makes it important to examine the contributions made by different people to preschoolers' emotion understanding. Obviously, young children glean unique information about emotions from the experiences of themselves and others. Varied sources of emotional understanding add to children's accumulating information.

## What Causes One's Own Emotions?

Young children begin to realize that the causes of an emotion can vary depending on who is experiencing it, and that potential elicitors have uniquely individual effects. One child is saddened by seeing her mother leave for work, but another becomes sad when someone wrecks his Legos. Vegetables for dinner cause one child's happiness, whereas another registers disgust (see "Use of Personalized Information," below).

Preschoolers are able to talk about what would make them happy, sad, angry, and afraid, especially when encouraged to do so within the context of playing with puppets. When an examiner says, "This puppet is so-oo sad . . . Let's pretend it is *you*. What would make you feel this way?", children often identify with the puppet (Denham & Zoller, 1991). Their conceptions of the causes of their own emotions are more complete than those they give for either peers or parents (Dunn & Hughes, 1998). They ascribe different causes to different emotions as well. That is, in our research we have found that children often cite nonsocial events for their happiness, such as playing with toys; social causes for their sadness and anger, such as wanting Mom and being punched, respectively; and fantasy causes for their fear, such as seeing a dinosaur. These results are largely consonant with those of Strayer's (1986) investigation, although we have studied even younger children within the preschool age range.

## What Causes Peers' Emotions?

Preschoolers have also been interviewed about their peers' naturally occurring emotions (Dunn & Hughes, 1998; Fabes et al., 1988, 1991). As with their own emotions, young children are able to perceive and report on a variety of causes for peers' emotions. They refer to social, nonsocial, and internal causes for displays of happiness, sadness, anger, and distress. For example, nonsocial reasons for happiness, sadness, and anger, respectively, include "A sunny day," "Something is broken," and "Watching the news on TV." In contrast, social reasons given for these same emotions include "Playing with friends/me," "Her dad spanks her," and "Someone doesn't do what he wants," respectively. Importantly, the causes given for their peers' emotions often parallel those given by adults who have also witnessed the peers' displays (Fabes et al., 1988). Thus children and adults both rely on context—namely, events that are actually taking place—to accurately determine causes of anger and distress.

Children, like adults, are also sensitive to internal causes of others' emotions (see also Stein & Trabasso, 1989). When intense emotions are displayed, children are more likely to focus on internal factors associated with the target child's goals. In describing the cause of a peer's intense anger, a preschooler says, "He wanted his block tower to stay up," instead of "She knocked down his block tower."

Even more importantly, preschoolers focus on different internal states for their peers' differing emotions (Denham & Zoller, 1991; Fabes et al., 1988). Children most often supply social reasons for anger, sadness, and distress or pain. Physical and material interactions with other people, such as being punched or having a toy taken away, are often noted. This finding is not surprising, given the frequency of conflict in peer play.

It is understandable that preschoolers may cite similar themes and persons as causes for anger and sadness (although some researchers report more differentiated responses; see Dunn & Hughes, 1998). Both emotions can result from the same events, with anger evolving from a focus on the other person's obstructing one's goal, and sadness from a more solitary focus on the unachieved goal state (Fabes et al., 1988). With respect to happiness, children often give social physical, verbal, and nonverbal causes, such as being tickled, getting a compliment, or making a funny face. They also cite impersonal contexts to explain happiness, such as having a big playroom full of toys (Strayer, 1986).

But children do find it trickier to discern the causes of peers' happiness and sadness than to identify the causes of their anger or pain. In fact, even though children are most accurate in identifying the *existence* of happiness, they are least accurate in identifying *causes* of happiness. Most findings suggest that children are more successful in identifying causes of negative emotions (Dunn & Hughes, 1998; Fabes et al., 1991). Others' happiness and sadness can be less powerful and salient than their anger and distress. A peer's smile, or a friend's tears as he or she huddles alone, can be powerful social communicators; most children would be able to identify the feelings expressed. But a response to these emotions is not almost mandatory, as it is to a friend who pushes another in anger, or to a child who falls off the jungle gym and screams in pain. Others' anger and distress may produce more threatening and adverse consequences, so that it is adaptive for children to be more attentive to and concerned with these emotions and their causes. Moreover, peers' happiness and sadness also may be more abstract and complex than their anger and distress, because they are more often internally caused (Fabes et al., 1991).

Children become more able to understand the causal complexities of emotion throughout the preschool period. Through their increased social sensitivity and experience, older preschoolers are also developing more strategies for appraising others' emotions when available cues are less salient and consensual. Five-year-olds are more likely than 3- and 4-year-olds to focus their explanations of emotions on personal dispositions as opposed to goal states: "She had a bad day," instead of "She didn't want Billy to play with her."

Hence, older preschoolers' descriptions of the causes of emotions are becoming more abstract and less idiosyncratic than younger preschoolers' (Fabes et al., 1991). Obviously, this reasoning can be much more useful in actual interaction with friends. I will address this important corollary of preschoolers' growing understanding of emotions more comprehensively in Chapter 6.

Finally, although both girls and boys develop understanding of the causes of emotions during the preschool years, they sometimes have differing foci. Girls sometimes cite more interpersonal causes of emotion, presumably because of their experience in relationships and their reasoning about the social world (Fabes et al., 1988; Strayer, 1986).

## What Causes Parents' Emotions?

Over and above the unique emotional information that different relationship partners provide, the very nature of the parent–child relationship puts a spotlight on parents' emotions. Not only are parents' emotional displays ubiquitous in children's daily lives (Patterson, 1980), but children are also motivated to understand feelings in such an important relationship. Parents are special social partners: They are in a position of authority, so that children are likely to attend to their emotions and want to please them. At the same time, parents tend to be clear and emphatic in their displays of emotions around their children, for both strategic and didactic reasons. Parents' emotions are likely to differ in some important ways from those of peers and of children themselves. Consequently, children learn a great deal about the causes and consequences of emotions from their parents.

Children aged 4 and 5 can demonstrate coherent understanding of the differing causes for parental happiness, sadness, and anger. Children assessed via their play actions and verbalizations during a semistructured dollhouse play interview do not see themselves as causing a majority of parental emotions (Denham, 1996a; see also Dunn & Hughes, 1998). Preschoolers comprehend that a variety of circumstances and events can cause their parents' emotions, in contrast with children assessed with predominantly verbal procedures (as in Covell & Abramovitch, 1987, 1988).

The overall pattern of our research findings is qualified, however. First, preschoolers, especially 3-year-olds, still have a good bit of difficulty specifying causes of parental sadness and anger; about 30% of all preschool participants give no causes or uncodable ones (compared to 40% "don't know" responses from 4- to 5-year-olds on Dunn & Hughes's verbal measure). Second, preschoolers, especially boys, do see themselves as causing *mothers'*, but not fathers', emotions. Given the sometimes confrontational and sometimes lighthearted nature of children's interactions with their mothers, this assumption on their part is not entirely egocentric. Preschoolers *do* cause a lot of happiness, anger, and distress for their mothers!

In general, however, young children can give specific causes for particular parental emotions. Their causal conceptions are well articulated and even poignant, corresponding with culturally understood scenarios. They are often able to enumerate causes that fit into categories, as they do for their own and their peers' emotions—social and nonsocial physical, social control, social verbal, social and nonsocial material, and nonsocial events. Table 3.1 depicts some of their descriptions. Most also dovetail with causes of their own emotions given by children in other studies (e.g., Covell & Abramovitch, 1987; Dunn & Hughes, 1998).

*Summary*

Thus, young children are processing even relatively fine nuances about the emotion–event linkages in their daily lives. Although the categories children use to understand their own, their peers', and their parents' emotions are similar, the actual content of the scenarios they describe for each often differ. They say, "He's feeling mean," or "Daddy yelled at her," to describe a parent's anger. In contrast, they say, "Billy took Mike's Power Ranger," or "My brother called me names and Mommy said I couldn't hit him," to talk about themselves or peers. Furthermore, as might be expected, their explanations of the causes of emotions are most adequate when referring to themselves rather than to their peers or parents (Dunn & Hughes, 1998). These distinctions amid similarities prompt a search for the logical foundations of young children's solid understanding of emotions.

**TABLE 3.1.** Examples of Children's Conceptions of the Causes of Parents' Emotions

Causes of happiness

*Social nonverbal:* "Neighbors moved in," "The boy's cleaning up the mess," "I love him."
*Social verbal:* "I told him something funny," "Mommy says 'I love you.' "
*Nonsocial events:* "She took a nice bath," "She likes cooking dinner."
*Social physical:* "Because I gave her a kiss, a hug," "I tickled his back."
*Social control:* "Because I didn't bother her," "Because I eat all my supper."
*Social material:* "How about we go to the store and buy Mom stockings! Yeah! Buy her high-heeled shoes!"
*Nonsocial material:* "She has a teddy bear," "He has lots of candy."

Causes of sadness

*Nonsocial physical:* "He fell down," "She fell off the roof," "She wants a baby."
*Social physical:* "Someone hit her," "I kicked him," "I fell down."
*Social nonverbal:* "When a stranger comes," "Daddy's/Mommy's angry."
*Nonsocial material:* "Something broke," "The sink won't work," "We have no sandwich."
*Nonsocial events:* "Maybe he got in jail," "Because she had to move to a new house."

Causes of anger

*Social verbal:* "They're fighting over whose turn it was to cook dinner."
*Social control:* "Because I ran away," "Because I go to bed with gum in my mouth."
*Social physical/internal:* "Brother hit sister," "I spanked him," "Daddy pushed Mom."
*Nonsocial physical/internal:* "He's feeling mean," "He's had a bad day," "Maybe she sat on wet paint."
*Nonsocial events:* "He drove to the zoo and back and got mad at everybody," "She almost got run over."

*Note.* From Denham (1996a).

# Explaining Children's Understanding of the Causes of Emotion

What is the basis of children's early comprehension of the causes of emotion? How does this understanding develop? Currently there are three models that address young children's causal reasoning about emotions. These are prototype, event structure, and desire–belief analyses. Descriptions of each and an attempt at synthesis follow.

## Prototype Approach

A "prototype" describes general types of events that correlate with specific emotions; it links emotion and the common situations that cause it. Children aged 4 to 12, when interviewed and asked to tell what would make them happy, mad, sad, and scared, gave elements of adult emotion prototypes (Harter & Whitesell, 1989; Whitesell, 1989). Table 3.2 depicts the prototypical events that preschoolers think cause emotions, along with specific examples of each. These prototypes make it dear that even 4-year-olds know a lot about the typical causes of emotions.

But the specific prototype exemplars provided by children at different ages reflect age-appropriate content that are not usually found in the reports of adults; most adults, for instance, no longer consider the fearful possibility of tigers in the house. And not all features of prototypes available to older children and adults are necessarily in place among younger children. Preschoolers are likely to give one or a few very concrete causal examples of an emotion within one particular prototypical category. If asked, "What made you sad?", a preschooler can probably give an answer referring to harm to the self: "I got a boo-boo on my knee." In contrast, older children can give multiple examples within a single prototype. In talking about harm to the self, an older child reports all of the following: "I got hurt on the play-

**TABLE 3.2.** Prototypical Causes of Basic Emotions, with Quotes from Children

| Emotion | Causal event (general) | Example (specific) |
|---------|------------------------|--------------------|
| Happiness | Pleasurable stimuli | Tickling, a kiss |
| Happiness | Getting or doing something desired | Playing with dolls, Daddy coming home, a birthday present |
| Sadness | Harm to self | "Daniel hits me," falling off the bike |
| Sadness | Loss of a relationship | Someone won't play |
| Sadness | Undesirable events | Moving to a new house |
| Sadness | Powerlessness | Having a bad dream |
| Anger | Physical harm | "Bullies fight with me," being bitten by a baby sister |
| Anger | Psychological harm | Being made to eat liver, having a block tower knocked down, "Someone hurt my feelings" |
| Anger | Something not working, insurmountable obstacles | "My toys wore out," "I didn't get my way" |
| Fear | Anticipated harm | "I thought tigers were in my room", "Monsters were going to gobble me up" |
| Fear | Unfamiliar situations | Being left alone |

*Note.* Data from Denham and Zoller (1991).

ground," "My best friend said something mean to me," and "I was sick last week and couldn't breathe." Still older children and adults show an even more abstract understanding of the general prototype categories. They ask themselves, "What makes me sad?", and then answer, "When something happens to hurt me in any way."

In essence, the prototype approach characterizes the social cognition of emotions by referring to clusters of exemplars that share specific meanings and themes. Young children begin to grasp the thematic ideas by using the perspective of their own limited experiences. Caregivers' awareness of these themes, and of young children's capacity to comprehend them, can be useful.

> When Joelle says she is sad because she had an argument with her sister, her mother can empathize and make helpful suggestions, because she has felt the same way after arguments. In contrast, a day care provider may have no idea what Martin is talking about when he asserts, "I'm mad because I missed the snow." Nonetheless, an astute caregiver who can discern the theme of "things not working" can engage Martin in a more fruitful discussion to help him manage his feelings and become positively involved in play.

## Event Structure Approach

Whereas the prototype approach encompasses emotional themes, the event structure model focuses on processes—on the changes in goal states that result in emotion. The emphasis is on the information-processing steps that are taken to come to an experience of emotion, and especially on the goals that are operative when emotions are elicited by events. The details of the "story" behind the experience of emotion are not crucial elements, as they are in prototype theory.

Event structure analyses are useful because they capture the processes children use to determine the causes and consequences of happiness, sadness, anger, and fear (Stein & Jewett, 1986; Stein & Levine, 1989, 1990; Stein & Trabasso, 1989; see Chapter 2). For happiness, four causal dimensions exist. First, children must perceive some aspect of the event as novel with respect to the ability to maintain, attain, or avoid a particular goal state. Next, they must infer that a valued state has been achieved. In other words, children must realize that something new has happened, and that because of it, something good will happen or something bad will be avoided. Then children must realize that attaining or maintaining the goal has a high probability. Last, they need to recognize that the enjoyment of the goal state or goal maintenance will follow the event's outcome. A child reasons that getting candy will lead to happiness because a valued state has been achieved, and will no doubt be enjoyable.

In contrast, both anger and sadness can occur (or co-occur) because of loss and aversive states, by failure to attain a goal state that is wanted or failure to avoid the unwanted. The causal dimensions for sadness include novelty, inferences that a valued state is not achieved and cannot be reinstated, and a belief that the goal will not be enjoyed. One preschooler may reason that another child is sad because his mother has left him at the day care center, even though he wished and expected to stay with her, and that his valued state of "staying with Mommy" is not achieved. When this child cries and cries, the other child may reason that the child who is crying wants his mother even though he cannot rejoin her now.

In anger, children focus on the conditions that cause the failure to attain a wanted state or avoid an unwanted one; they respond to the loss or aversive state by inferring that the obstructed goal can be reinstated. Then, as a consequence of anger, they may enact a plan to reinstate the goal. Hence, a child may reason that anther child is angry because he did not get to keep all the blocks and is fighting to get them back.

In fear, children are aware that maintaining a desired state is now very unlikely. Their attention is focused on the cause of this probable failure to maintain the desired state and the consequences of it. For instance, on seeing a boy crying and backing up at the top of the slide on the playground, a preschool girl may reason that the boy thinks he is probably going to fall, and that he is hanging on tight to keep this from happening so he won't get hurt.

Even 3-year-olds can judge the causes and consequences of emotions, using the two sources of information critical to event analyses. They recognize internal goals, such as wanting to keep a toy, and external outcomes, such as losing a toy. Reasoning from these premises helps them differentiate emotional possibilities. They distinguish fear from anger and sadness by the external outcome expected, associating anticipation of harm only with fear. Those who express sadness over an obstacle in their way, instead of anger, focus on the permanent, irreparable loss of the goal. In a more abstract sense, when children of this age are deciding how they would feel in a situation, they seem to use the two necessary conditions for distinguishing among emotions (Stein & Jewett, 1986; Stein & Levine, 1989): (1) the goals of wanting/having, versus not wanting/not having, states; and (2) the outcomes inherent in the certainty or uncertainty of attaining these internal states.

*Desire-Belief Approach*

Although the language of the models differs, the desire–belief approach actually shares its emphasis on beliefs and desires with the event structure model. What the person in an emotion-eliciting situation *wants* is key. Children between the ages of 3 and 6 become significantly more accurate and consistent in understanding that emotional reactions depend on both desire and belief (Harris, 1989, 1993; Lagattuta, Wellman, & Flavell, 1997). Very young children base their reasoning about the cause of happiness on their awareness that being pleased or happy is a function of the match between desire and reality, such as when they receive a gift (Hadwin & Perner, 1991). That is, happiness occurs when actors anticipate getting what they desire (Harris, 1989).

Along with their understanding of desire-dependent emotions, children as young as 3 years of age also comprehend belief-dependent emotions, such as surprise (Wellman & Banerjee, 1991). If a preschool girl *believes* she is staring at a large decorative block, and suddenly a boy bursts from his hiding place within his box, the discrepancy between her belief and reality cause her surprise. In this case, surprise occurs when what the girl expects or believes does *not* happen. It is important to note that even though preschoolers accurately report this false-belief basis for surprise, they also report surprise when they merely gain knowledge where they were previously ignorant (Ruffman & Keenan, 1996). They do not merely understand the simple links between various situations and associated emotions, but are already capable of more abstract conceptions (Wellman & Banerjee, 1991).

*Integrating the Three Models*

The three approaches to explaining children's causal understanding of emotions are all persuasive, but their proponents consider each to be unique and to have more explanatory power than the others. Stein and Trabasso (1989) assert that the information-processing focus inherent in the event structure perspective is incompatible with a prototype approach, and Harter and Whitesell (1989) are similarly discouraging from their opposing viewpoint.

Even so, a rapprochement among the approaches can be proposed. A synthesis of viewpoints describes children's means of understanding their emotional world better than any single perspective does. Perhaps the event structure (novelty suspending ongoing thoughts, the wanting–not wanting and having/not having goal states, and the certainty of attaining or maintaining these states) may actually overarch prototypical examples, or form their logical basis. That is, event prototype exemplars may provide the thematic content of the event schema (see also Fischer et al., 1989). To paraphrase Stein and Trabasso (1989), both the underlying concept structure of the event, and the event itself, are important aspects of preschoolers' knowledge of emotions.

Distinguishing emotions both by event structure, and by thematic similarities among the events that cause them and the consequences that ensue, is important. We (Denham & Zoller, 1991) and Fabes et al. (1988, 1991) used both approaches, and the results are consistent with Harter & Whitesell's (1989), Whitesell's (1989), and Stein and Trabasso's (1989) analyses. It seems reasonable that we need to know both how a child is reasoning and what the child is reasoning about, so that we have a clear picture of development from either theoretical or practical standpoints.

This synthesis of approaches, as illustrated in Figure 3.1, adds to our understanding of the reasoning both children and adults go through when trying to make sense of their emotional world. Knowing the "how" of children's thinking about emotions can help caregivers comprehend their own children's sometimes idiosyncratic reasoning, and assist them in intervening to aid in affect regulation.

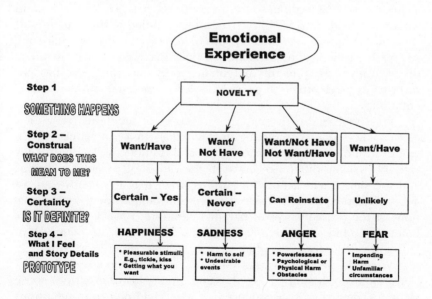

FIGURE 3.1. Resolving the event structure and prototype analyses of emotions' causes.

*Alex's preschool teacher, seeing his angry face, may accurately infer that he is focused on something he wants but does not have. She has isolated the important aspects of the event–goal and outcome. But what exactly is his goal, and what is the problematic outcome that's making him mad? Accordingly, her understanding of the event could prompt her to pinpoint the prototypical source of Alex's anger–his friend's misdeed. Alex considers that his friend "stole" the blocks, even without realizing that Alex considered them "his." Focusing again on Alex's goal, his teacher can also predict that he will probably swing into unbridled action to get the blocks back. Clearly, Alex can profit from his teacher's assistance on the "how" and the "what" of his emotional event. She can help him, first to refrain from hurting his friend, and then to reconstrue the whole event.*

The cognitive information processing that takes place during appraisals of emotional experience (see Chapter 1, Figure 1.1) may proceed according to an event or desire–belief formula, but may be *about* prototypical experiences that happen often to people of all ages.

## Understanding the Consequences of Emotions

Children use their recognition of the consequences of emotions in their behavioral decision making, just as they use their comprehension of the causes of emotions. Discerning consequences of emotion can help a child know what to do in social situations, such as "How do I respond when my friend is mad?" In fact, an understanding of the outcomes of their own emotions, and the reactions of others, may form the substrate of preschoolers' responses to emotions in general (whether sympathetic or insensitive). Despite this potential importance, this topic has not received as much attention as preschoolers' knowledge of the *causes* of emotion.

Preschoolers can distinguish the causes of emotions from their consequences when completing stories about why a protagonist felt an emotion, and what the protagonist did as a result (Russell, 1990). They can also tell the difference between the causes of parental emotions and the subsequent actions of parents when they felt happy, sad, or angry (Denham, 1996a). Table 3.3 depicts examples of their explanations of the consequences of parental emotions. Clearly, preschoolers hold some quite accurate ideas about the behavioral consequences of emotion—what people do when they experience different emotions.

What do people do as a consequence of someone else's emotions? In a recent study, I asked 4- and 5-year-olds to enact dollhouse vignettes depicting consequences of the children's own emotions (Denham, 1997). Children attributed plausible, nonrandom parental reactions to their own emotions. They saw their parents as matching

**TABLE 3.3.** Examples of Children's Conceptions of the Consequences of Their Own Emotions

Means of expressing happiness

*Shared activities*: "He dances," "She makes a pie," "She would buy things for us."

Means of expressing sadness

*Withdrawal*: "He goes to sleep," "She lays in her bed."

*Other*: "She went to the doctor," "Daddy wants a new kid."

Means of expressing anger

*Negative expression*: "She goes and breaks all the furniture," "He gives spankings," "Daddy goes out the door, bye-bye, and SLAM!"

*Note.* From Denham (1996a).

their own happiness or reacting in an irrelevant way to it; performing pragmatic action after sadness or punishing a sibling who caused it; punishing anger; and comforting, acting to alleviate, or discussing a fear-eliciting stimulus. Parents were seen as unlikely to comfort happiness, to perform pragmatic helpful action after anger, to punish happiness or fear, or to match any negative emotion. Taken together, my investigations suggest that preschoolers have fairly solid conceptions of how even adults behave after experiencing their own emotional arousal, and of the specific responsiveness of caregivers to child emotions. So they are beginning to understand the behavioral consequences of emotions for both themselves and others. Children who understand what happens when emotions are experienced are better equipped to regulate their own emotions and react to those of others. More work is needed to plumb the limits and correlates of this consequential understanding.

## Relations between Emotional Expressiveness and Basic Understanding of Emotions

If children between 2 and 5 years old are acquiring such a solid corpus of basic emotion understanding, do any other aspects of emotional competence contribute to it? Importantly, children's own patterns of expressiveness contribute to this basic understanding of emotions. They need to experience moderate levels of a variety of emotions in order to construct social scripts about emotions. Preschoolers first reflect on and make judgments about their own emotions, and then generalize these judgments to others' feelings (Smiley & Huttenlocher, 1989). Even infants clearly experience positive affect sharing and distress relief. Given this experience of their own emotions, then, it is not surprising that toddlers evidence comprehension of happy–not happy states so very early.

Following Smiley and Huttenlocher's reasoning, overall expressiveness should contribute to understanding of emotion. I have found this to be true: Children who show more emotions during free play are more adept at understanding both emotional expressions and situations (e.g., Denham, 1986).

Second, the particular emotions children express and their social cognition about emotions also are related. Overall emotional security can contribute to emotion understanding (see Cummings, 1995a); children whose own emotional needs are met, and who feel generally happier, are more able to contemplate emotional issues. Again, my early work (Denham, 1986) supported this prediction: Children who were more emotionally positive showed greater comprehension of basic emotional expressions, and situations. Conversely, preschoolers who experienced much negative emotion (sadness, anger, or pain) were less able to focus on emotional experiences in order to acquire this basic-level knowledge.

But relations among aspects of emotionality and understanding of emotions are not quite this simple. The experience of at least *some* negative emotion is necessary for children to understand feelings. Children who more often experience anger and fear are also more fluent in verbally enumerating causes for these emotions than are children who rarely experience them (Denham & Zoller, 1990). Thus, parents and caregivers need to take into account their children's expressiveness patterns when trying to appreciate, or facilitate, the children's ability to comprehend emotions. Allowing children to experience emotions rather than suppressing them, encouraging positive emotion, and assisting them in their experience of negative emotion are important socialization themes, to which I will return in Chapter 4.


## USING EMOTION LANGUAGE

### Development in Patterns of Emotion Language Use

Young children do converse about emotions, although such conversation is a small portion of their entire discourse. They show substantial ability to use emotion-descriptive adjectives, and to understand these terms when used by adults (Bretherton et al., 1986; Ridgeway & Kuczaj, 1985). Even very young children refer to internal emotional states (e.g., distress, pain, joy, anger) and to their causes and consequences. During their second and third years, toddlers begin to employ emotion language to influence others to meet their own emotional needs (Dunn, Brown, & Beardsall, 1991). They use emotion words to obtain comfort, support, or attention ("I cried in bed"); to express pleasure or affection ("Give me a kiss! I love you!"); to maintain a happy state ("I like this merry-go-round!"); or to anticipate, achieve, or avoid other affective states ("No *Jurassic Park* movie; too scary").

Over 75% of 3-year-old children use terms for feeling good, happy, sad, afraid, angry, loving, mean, and surprised (Ridgeway & Kuczaj, 1985). By the end of the preschool period, over 75% of 6-year-olds also use terms for feeling comfortable, excited, upset, glad, unhappy, relaxed, bored, lonely, annoyed, disappointed, shy, pleased, worried, calm, embarrassed, hating, nervous, and cheerful (Ridgeway & Kuczaj, 1985). Finally, although kindergartners produce fewer synonyms for emotion words than grade school children do, they give similar proportions of synonyms across emotions (i.e., the largest variety of terms for happiness and sadness, and the fewest for guilt and pride; Whissell & Nicholson, 1991). Again, preschoolers show substantial understanding of emotion.

Preschoolers test and refine these understandings of emotional expressions, situations, causes, and consequences while talking with important persons in their lives. Emotion language "provides children with an especially powerful tool for understanding emotions" (Kopp, 1989, p. 349). They state their own feelings to people who need to know about them, obtain these persons' feedback about these feelings, and process causal associations between events and emotions.

*When Anson says, "I hate it when Daniel hits me all the time. It makes me really mad," his mother can sympathize and tell him it sounds as if he is justifiably offended. When he next asserts, in a puzzled voice, "But I don't know why he hits me. He never seems angry," his mother is then able to point out that Daniel indeed sounds unpredictable, and to help him decide what to do. Perhaps in his next encounter with Daniel, Anson can use emotion language directly in interpersonal negotiation to get the problem solved.*

## Using Emotion Language within the Family

As the example above suggests, young children do not construct their vocabulary of emotion in a nonsocial vacuum; other people participate. Over time, they have conversations about emotions with parents, grandparents, other caregivers, siblings, and peers (Bretherton & Beeghly, 1982; Bretherton et al., 1986; Howe, 1991; Shatz, 1994). Parental verbalizations about emotions undoubtedly assist young children in learning about expressing emotion and understanding emotions. Individual differences in mothers' usage of emotion language in its various functions give children unique understandings about emotion. (See Chapter 4 for an extended discussion of mothers' contribution to young children's use of emotion language within the family.)

Developmental changes can be discerned in the content and context of young children's feeling state talk (Brown & Dunn, 1991, 1992). Dunn and her associates have observed naturally occurring conversations about feelings between mothers and their 18- to 36-month-old children (Brown & Dunn, 1991, 1992; Dunn et al., 1987; Dunn & Munn, 1985). Children are not passive participants in such conversations. Between 24 and 36 months of age (Brown & Dunn, 1991), children refer to feeling states, and the content and context of emotion discourse both change. As toddlers near their third birthday, they begin to use emotion language in reflective discussions, especially about the causes and consequences of feeling states ("I miss Mom-Mom, I get sad"); as a means of manipulating the feelings and behaviors of others ("Talk nice, Mommy, don't be so mad"); and even in teasing (R: "I'm going to eat you all up! And I'll tell Grandpa you died." G: "You will! And will he be happy or sad?" R: "Sad.") (Shatz, 1994).

Thus, young children and their mothers use emotion language to fulfill a variety of functions, including socialization, explaining, guiding behavior, and questioning (Bretherton et al., 1986). When 3- and 4-year-olds talked with their mothers about photographs of infants expressing peak emotional expressions, they averaged almost one emotion term per photo (Denham, Cook, & Zoller, 1992). During their conversation, the function of children's emotion language was not simply to comment on the pictures ("He's crying"). They also used emotion words to explain causes ("She's happy because she likes her mom") to infer consequences ("If you were sad, I would ask Daddy to hug you") to ask questions about the infants' emotions ("He's making a sad face—what's the matter?"), and to guide another's behavior ("He's sad, he needs his mommy"). The variety of linguistic functions young children use in their conversations is testimony to their motivation to discuss emotional issues, and to their considerable body of knowledge about emotion.

Between 33 and 47 months of age, mother–child conversations about feelings decrease in frequency, whereas those between siblings increase, reflecting the increased ability of a younger sibling to engage in emotion conversation independent of the mother (Brown & Dunn, 1992). As interaction partners, older siblings are very different from mothers; they give preschoolers a new set of experiences in the use of emotion language. They are less likely to view their younger siblings' edification as a goal, less apt to be patient, and less able to "scaffold" conversations so that younger siblings can keep up. Not surprisingly, they focus more often on seeing that their own needs are met and talk more about their own feelings than mothers do, perhaps pushing their younger sibling to take their perspective (Brown & Dunn, 1992). Hence, emotion conversations with older siblings serve different functions than those with mothers do.

Preschool-age siblings, especially those who are good perspective takers, sometimes do use language to focus on their toddler siblings' emotions, particularly during maternal absences, conflicts, or play. Such use of emotion language allows older siblings to regulate interactions with toddlers, and to construct shared meanings about their world (Howe, 1991). An older sibling says, "You'd better stop that before you make me mad!" to regulate interaction, or "It made me cry, too, when I hit my head. Do you need Mom?" to construct shared meanings about caregiving. Siblings also engage in emotion talk centered on themes of play and humor, building complex shared jokes and pretense narratives.

These naturalistic investigations of conversations about emotions convincingly demonstrate toddlers' and preschoolers' increasing understanding of the emotional scripts of their cultures (Brown & Dunn, 1991, 1992; Dunn et al., 1987). It should also be noted that the family conversations transcribed by Dunn and colleagues contain much self-referential feeling state language used even by *very* young children; this calls into question the notion that the self-awareness of young children is severely limited. Caregivers and parents can capitalize on this ability, sensitively discussing the child's own experience.

## MORE SOPHISTICATED UNDERSTANDING OF OTHERS' EMOTIONAL EXPERIENCE

Sometimes knowing about emotion vocabulary, expressions of emotions, emotion-eliciting situations, and even the causes and consequences of emotions is not enough to permit an individual to interpret the emotional signals of others accurately. Information specific to a particular person in a particular situation may be needed. In a series of thought-provoking inquiries, Gnepp and colleagues have used a processing model to describe the information needed in deciding what emotion another person is experiencing or will experience in a given situation (Gnepp, 1983, 1989a, 1989b; Gnepp & Chilamkurti, 1988; Gnepp & Gould, 1985; Gnepp, Klayman, & Trabasso, 1982; Gnepp, McKee, & Domanic, 1987). Important elements in processing emotional information are (1) whether the situation is equivocal (i.e., whether it could elicit more than one emotion); (2) whether there are conflicting cues in the person's expressive patterns and the situation; and (3) whether personalized information is needed.

## Equivocal Situations

To identify the emotion another person is showing, the first question is whether the situation has a single strong emotional determinant common across persons. Young children are clearly capable of such determinations, as shown in my own group's work and that of Gnepp, Stein, and their colleagues (see also Borke, 1971). They imagine how they themselves would feel or how people in general feel in such situations.

But some situations do not have a strong emotion–event association. Different people feel different emotions in response to some emotion-eliciting events. One child is happy to encounter a large, friendly-looking dog, panting and "smiling" with mouth open. Another child is terrified in the same situation. More personal information is needed in order to know how the person is feeling.

Preschoolers are becoming aware that specialized information is sometimes needed to interpret emotions. They are beginning to recognize the equivocality inherent in some emotion situations—that is, the fact that some situations commonly elicit different emotional reactions in different people. We showed children a puppet showing an emotion contrasting with the child's own likely emotion, in vignettes designed to be equivocal; each child's job was to hold his or her own likely emotion in abeyance and to pick the correct emotion for the puppet (Denham & Couchoud, 1990a). For example, if a mother reported that a child was happy to go swimming, the puppet enacted fear.

The children in the study struggled to make such specialized inferences, but they were able to do so more frequently than expected by chance. They were most successful when positive and negative emotions were contrasted, rather than two negative emotions. Thus, they were often able to comprehend and indicate that the puppet was sad to go to preschool when they themselves would be happy. Even making these inferences required some effort, however.

> *Toma looked mystified while applying the happy face, correctly, on a puppet anticipating an oatmeal breakfast made by the mommy puppet. Personally, Toma would be angry about–in fact, would hate–an oatmeal breakfast. After he secured the puppet's happy face, he started talking rapidly to it: "I'd be mad! Oatmeal is yucky. It gets lumps, it's cold, it has no taste!"*

Assessing equivocality *and* differentiating between the more troublesome negative emotions was a task burden, so that choosing between two negative emotions was much more difficult than choosing between happiness and one negative emotion. Preschoolers struggled with situations that pitted two equally plausible negative emotions, as when the puppet was angry at anticipating punishment, instead of fearful as they themselves would be. In agreement with earlier results, error analyses indicated that vignettes involving fear, and to some extent anger, were the most difficult for the children to interpret.

In the same vein as my studies, Gnepp et al. (1987) told children stories describing different situations, some unequivocal and some equivocal. The children were asked to say they were thinking of only one feeling if they were sure how the protagonist felt, but to say they were thinking of two feelings if two were possible. Spontaneously acknowledging equivocality by saying that they were thinking of two feelings for vignettes, such as a dog's walking down the street toward the protagonist, was difficult for them. After these free responses, however, the experimenter probed for more information. When questioned about the dog vignette, many 5- and 6-year-olds were able to say, "Some kids like dogs and some don't," thereby acknowledging that equivocality exists. This task may have underestimated preschoolers' knowledge of equivocality. Gnepp et al. unwittingly were also asking children to acknowledge simultaneity/ambivalence of emotions, and thus were mingling two difficult areas of emotion understanding.

In sum, research suggests that preschoolers are beginning to deal with equivocality, especially if the necessary personalized inferences fit with their earliest distinctions among emotions—"good" feelings versus "bad" feelings, and among "bad" feelings, sadness and anger. For the preschoolers in Gnepp et al.'s (1987) study, the notion of equivocality was just emerging, whereas in our work (Denham & Couchoud, 1990a), preschoolers seemed to be further along in dealing with it. Methodological differences often fuel such discrepancies; as seen in myriad other areas, preschoolers' competence to differentiate equivocal emotional situations can be concealed by performance issues in tasks that require more than the children can give.

## Conflicting Expressive and Situational Cues to a Person's Emotion

Even if there is a strong emotion–event association in a situation, the person experiencing the event may react atypically. For instance, a person may smile when seeing a spider dropping into the room on a strand of web. Personal information is needed, then, not only when a situation is emotionally equivocal but also when an emotional reaction is atypical. However, interpreting a reaction as atypical requires a rather sophisticated decision—namely, *resolving* conflicting expressive and situational cues to emotions, rather than relying on one cue or the other.

The view that sources of emotional information are resolvable is a new one. This perspective stands in contrast to the long-standing debate about age changes in the relative weights children assign to facial and situational information about emotion. As early as 1979, Abramovitch and Daly asserted that 4-year-olds can decode the emotional aspects of the facial expressions of a wide range of stimulus persons, such as classmates, unfamiliar peers, and adults. Furthermore, they contended, this expression identification increasingly enables children to recognize the emotional content of situations. This reasoning seems plausible, although the converse could be equally true: Children may take in the expressions common across certain situations and recognize them as angry, for example.

Such interconnection between expressions and situations is almost unavoidable. But which type of cue is most important in children's judgments as they become more emotionally competent? Situational cues may become more important than expression in discerning how someone *really* feels, as children begin to understand the salience of display rules. But expression may also become more important as children become more sensitive to the equivocality of situations (Gnepp, 1989a). The question of whether facial or situational information is primary may be unresolvable.

Perhaps a more fruitful line of inquiry would involve the assumption that both sorts of information are important, with the weight given each in specific contexts most illuminating. Children may learn to weight each source of emotional information strategically, much as they come to utilize multiple sources of information in cognitive tasks, such as balance scale problems (Richards & Siegler, 1981; Siegler & Jenkins, 1989). This possibility is especially credible because cognitive/linguistic ability has been related to emotion knowledge, as indexed both by talking about emotion and by the results of our puppet measures (Denham & Couchoud, 1990a, 1990b, 1991; Denham, Zoller, & Couchoud, 1994; Smith & Walden, in press).

The relative weights preschoolers assign to expressive and situational cues of emotions were examined, using a series of pictures in which facial and situational information were conflicting (Hoffner & Badzinski, 1989). Children indicated the type (happy or sad) and intensity of each character's emotion. Reliance on situational information increased with age from preschool to fifth grade, and reliance on facial information decreased after the preschool period. Children's ability to resolve conflicting information also increased with age. Thus, the relative influence of situational and expressive information on 4- through 8-year-olds' emotion recognition shows a developmental trend, from noticing only one type of information to considering both expressive and situational evidence (Wiggers & Van Lieshout, 1985). When situational and expressive indicators are discrepant (suggesting differing emotions), young, concrete thinkers infer the most recognizable, simplest emotion, rather than relying solely on either type of information. This pattern can be expected, as children's abilities to decenter and examine multiple sources of information increase through the preoperational and concrete operational periods.

The valences of expressions and situations probably make a difference, too. At all age levels in the Hoffner and Badzinski (1989) study, children were less able to resolve an anomalous positive expression paired with a negative situation (e.g., smiling while getting an injection) than a negative expression paired with a positive situation (e.g., crying at a birthday party). They could conceive of masking an emotion or substituting one emotion for another in a negative situation less readily than they could envision the extenuating reasons for feeling bad during a normally pleasant time (see also Gnepp, 1983).

To describe *how* children weigh sources of emotional information, Gove and Keating (1979) presented 3- and 5-year-olds with stories in which the outcome was the same for each character, but the facial expression of the characters differed. For example, in one story a child was happy to receive a dog as a gift, but in another the child was afraid. In one-third to one-half of the responses, these young subjects were able to explain the differences psychologically (*"She* likes dogs, but *he* is really scared of them"). They demonstrated an understanding that the same situation can give rise to different emotions, and thus expressions, in different people; they were weighing multiple sources of information. Children who could not give such sophisticated explanations demonstrated their inability to recognize that different people could feel different ways about the same situation. They tended to reconstruct the situation ("This dog doesn't have big teeth, so she likes him a lot").

Given vignettes involving only one person, rather than two persons in one situation (e.g., a girl smiling while getting an injection in the doctor's office), children told stories about conflicting facial and situational information (Gnepp, 1983). The 3- and 4-year-olds were able to reconcile the conflict to form a coherent explanation of the person's circumstances about half of the time, albeit by attributing an idiosyncratic perspective to the character ("She likes shots"). Such attribution of idiosyncrasy may be a precursor of understanding the psychological causes of personalized reactions to emotion-eliciting situations (Gnepp, 1983, 1989b). Some 3- and 4-year-olds gave even more elaborate explanations of idiosyncratic reactions in specific situations, often by introducing information that would change the character's emotion ("This is a special shot that won't hurt") (Gnepp, 1983). Such children are starting to see the personal complexity of even situations that appear, on the surface, emotionally unequivocal.

But even older preschoolers are often unable to ask spontaneous questions to help them resolve emotionally equivocal situations (Gould, 1984). Apparently they can sometimes use information about equivocal situations, but do not automatically search for it, or even notice that they need to do so. Many preschoolers are still working on the ability to recognize the complex details of differing perspectives—the fact that desires and goals often differ from person to person, and why. Sometimes they still prefer simple, script-based analyses of emotion. They may also have a vague notion, based on their experiences, that a person can encounter negative emotions within normally positive situations, but this knowledge is imperfect. Moreover, these youngsters may not have been exposed to display rules for substituting positive emotional expression in negative situations. Taken together, investigations reveal two major obstacles to a preschoolers' ability to create a sophisticated union of expressive and situational indicators of emotion: cognitive limitations and experiential/socialization limitations. Clearly, the ability to understand psychological causes of personalized emotional reactions is just emerging in some children during the preschool period.

## Use of Personalized Information

What kinds of personal information do preschoolers use in interpreting emotions? First, unique normative information is often important: "Sarah lives in Green Valley, where all the people are friendly with tigers and play games with them all the time" (Gnepp et al., 1982, p. 116). When asked what feelings Sarah would experience, preschoolers used unique normative information about liking tigers to modify their responses to a normally unequivocal situation. Preschoolers are also becoming aware that normative cultural categories such as age and gender moderate the emotions experienced in differing situations. For example, a boy may not be overjoyed to receive a doll as a gift.

Second, information about personality characteristics that are stable across time and situations can be especially useful. Gnepp and Chilamkurti (1988) told children stories in which the protagonist was honest, a clown, helpful, cruel, shy, or selfish. Even 6-year-old children used such information to answer questions about feelings in situations that normally could be considered unequivocal (e.g., how would a clown feel if he wore one black shoe and one white one to school, and everybody laughed?). No studies have examined use of personality characteristics to determine emotion in children younger than 6, so it is impossible to say when the ability first appears.

Third, immediately present person-specific information is sometimes needed. Gnepp et al. (1982) provided stories in which characters' behavioral dispositions modified normally strong emotion–event associations: "Mark eats grass whenever he can. It's dinnertime and Mother says they're having grass for dinner. How will Mark feel?" Children aged 4 and 5 utilized such information; their responses reflected the unique perspective of the story character ("Mark will be happy to have grass for dinner"). The children also gave more weight to such person-specific information than to normative information when the two kinds of information conflicted.

A fourth source of personalized information is an individual's past history. Young children use such information, but less frequently than adults do, because much inference is needed to coordinate it with the current emotional reaction. Gnepp and Gould (1985) told stories in which personalized information was embedded in descriptions of the person's past experiences: "Robin's best friend said she didn't like her any more. The next day, Robin saw her best friend on the playground. How did she feel?" Five-year-olds made more situational inferences ("Robin was happy to see her friend because they could play together") than personalized ones ("Robin felt sad because she knew her friend didn't like her any more"). Although older children made more personalized inferences in a condition where they asked to explain the character's atypical emotion (e.g., Robin's sadness at seeing her friend), kindergartners did not. Use of this type of personalized information is basically beyond them.

## Summary

Children in the preschool period are beginning to understand how the causes of an emotion can differ from person to person or from situation to situation. They are uniting expressions and situations in a more sophisticated way. Many complex judgments about emotions remain difficult, however. Understanding that young children cannot yet make these inferences is as important as knowing how proficient they are in many other areas of emotion understanding. A mother can't expect her 4-year-old son to comprehend completely the complex history of her personal aversion for chocolate ice cream. And a preschool girl's inability to refer in an abstract way to emotion-related aspects of her own personality accounts for her answer to the question "Why are you so mad?": "Because I am."

## BECOMING AWARE OF EMOTION REGULATION STRATEGIES

People experience emotion when valued goals have been either attained or thwarted. We feel happy when we get a present that we wanted, and sad when we fall off a new bicycle. The emotions that signal the attainment or thwarting of a goal act as intrapersonal regulators. When we feel negative emotions, we want to feel better; when we feel positive ones, we want to continue to feel good. We want to maintain or achieve a valued state and avoid an aversive state; we want to regulate our emotions. Young children are learning about strategies to regulate their own and others' emotions. That is, they are learning how to change emotions, both negative and positive (Stein & Levine, 1990).

### Ways to Change Negative Emotions

Young children are motivated to change certain emotions (Carlson, Felleman, & Masters, 1983). The simplest approach to accessing young children's ideas about changing emotions is to cite an emotion and ask them to tell or to act out how it could be changed. In line with what adults expect, they deem anger and sadness the most changeworthy, and happiness the least. In studies with various methodologies, preschoolers have shown that they comprehend specific nurturant and aggressive strategies to change sadness and anger, including physical, verbal, social, material, and helping–hindering strategies (Denham, 1996a; Fabes et al., 1988; Fabes & Eisenberg, 1992; McCoy & Masters, 1985). They cite physical and material strategies to remediate sadness, material and verbal strategies for anger, and verbal and physical strategies for distress; see Table 3.4 for quotations referring to changing their parents' negative emotions (Denham, 1996a). I found that the prevalent intervention for changing parental sadness or anger was nurturant physical ("Give a kiss/hug"). The youngsters knew that these are disarming, cheering strategies. For changing both sadness and anger, girls were more likely than boys to cite nurturant physical interventions (Denham, 1996a).

Another approach to examining children's strategies for changing emotions is to tell them story stems and ask how to aid the protagonist in changing emotion. Children aged 4 to 9 were told increasingly complex stories about losing a parent's radio, parents' anger after a bad day at work, or parents' arguing (Covell & Miles, 1992). All children said that the story child could change a parent's anger. This is a hopeful sign for families! But the youngest group cited more indirect means that did not address the cause of parents' emotion, such

**TABLE 3.4.** Examples of Children's Conceptions of Ways to Change Parents' Negative Emotions

Changing sadness

*Nurturant physical*: "Give a kiss/hug," "Rub his back."
*Nurturant material*: "Give her something to eat."
*Nurturant helping*: "Let her sleep," "Clean up the mess."
*Nurturant verbal*: "Say sorry."

Changing anger

*Nurturant physical*: "Give a kiss/hug."
*Nurturant material*: "Give him an apple."
*Nurturant helping*: "Clean up the house," "Not bother him."
*Nurturant verbal*: "Say 'Don't be mad, Mom,' " "Say 'I love you.' "

*Note.* From Denham (1996a).

as painting a parent a picture, doing well in school, or buying a parent a gift. Direct strategies were cited by the younger children only for the least complex story, where the problem was easily solved—getting another radio.

These indirect strategies may appear less useful on the surface, but in this case preschoolers may have shown unwitting wisdom. Another group of children and parents rated the actual effectiveness of these indirect and direct strategies. Both parents and children endorsed certain indirect strategies as *more* effective than direct ones (e.g., being good, smiling, showing affection). Other indirect strategies, such as doing well at school or buying a gift, were seen as less effective (cf. Denham, 1996a). In other words, children considered strategies that would generally elicit parental happiness to be effective in reducing parental anger. They thought that directly addressing the anger-producing stimulus would be less useful, maybe even risky. So, interestingly, the youngest children in Covell and Miles's first sample would have been most successful in alleviating parental anger. Even though they were required to answer verbally—a difficult mode of response for them—these young children knew how mothers' anger is best diffused. The older children's more direct, cognitively more adequate responses might have gotten them in trouble!

## Ways to Change Positive Emotions

Knowing what actions to avoid in order to maintain happiness and other positive states is important, too. Children know that material, social, and physical aggression can change happiness to negative affect (McCoy & Masters, 1985). In the Denham (1996a) study, the prevalent intervention to change parental happiness was antisocial physical means (e.g., the boy doll punches the father doll twice and says, "I'll kick your butt"). Preschoolers also know that a person feeling "just okay" will feel worse if exposed to material aggression and better if exposed to material/social nurturance.

Sometimes, however, preschoolers become confused when asked about changing happiness: Why would this ever be a goal? I found (Denham, 1996a) that girls, especially older ones, were more likely than boys to cite nurturant social means to change parental happiness. Often when giving such a response, children seemed puzzled, concretely assuming that if an emotion needed changing, then nurturance was called for. In general, preschool-age children find the idea of changing happiness somewhat outlandish.

## Cognitive Strategies for Changing Emotions

Young children have some ideas—rather effective ones at that—about changing their own and others' negative emotions. They are less skilled at how to change positive emotions. Over time, they come to understand that means of regulating emotions differ in effectiveness. Moreover, they are developing some more internal, mentalistic strategies to deal with emotions, especially negative ones. But these sophisticated means of changing emotion never predominate. In fact, cognitive strategies to change emotion are given less frequently than behavioral strategies across the whole age range of 4 to 15 years (Brown, Covell, & Abramovitch, 1991; see Chapter 5). So, although 4- to 6-year-olds recognize cognitive control strategies (e.g., remembering a happy time or telling yourself how to feel better) when reminded of them, they do not generate them on their own. This inability to generate strategies spontaneously is parallel to preschoolers' inability to take personalized information about emotion into account spontaneously, suggesting that less sophisticated cognitive development is the root of these limitations.

As I have argued previously, a more engaging methodology could more clearly elucidate preschoolers' strategies, even cognitive ones, for changing emotions. It would be specifically geared for maximizing the performance of preschoolers, with task demands tailored for the age range. In a study using such methods, 3- to 5-year-olds were presented with stories in which characters were experiencing sadness, anger, or fear. The stories were presented as puppet plays. The puppet's feelings were common to children's experience and were explicitly stated. For example, Jacob was angry because his teacher told him there wasn't enough time for his show and tell. He was very angry, but he wanted to enjoy his time at school and not feel so angry inside (see Banerjee

& Eggleston, 1993; see also Banerjee, 1997a, 1997b). Children did not have the added response burdens of independently inferring the character's emotion or of puzzling over the story. They were also engaged fully in pretend play with the puppet.

One group of children was asked to generate strategies for coping with the emotional situations presented in the stories. Another group was asked to choose from the following strategies:

- External strategies, such as changing the external situations, location, or emotional expression, or seeking external help (e.g., Jacob should put a smile on his face).
- Mentalistic strategies involving thought processes, such as redirecting thoughts, reinterpreting the situation, or engaging in pretense (e.g., Jacob should think about how much fun it will be to do his show and tell tomorrow).
- Ineffectual strategies that would not work, such as merely repeating the story facts, doing something that would exacerbate negative feelings, or simply accepting the emotion (e.g., Jacob should stay in class and just sit there).

In both methodologies, children reported effectual external or mentalistic strategies approximately 90% of the time. Furthermore, mentalistic strategies were reported at least once by half of the children in the open-ended group, and were chosen more often than ineffectual strategies in the forced-choice group. Even without benefit of forced-choice strategies, the oldest children in the open-ended group provided more mentalistic than ineffectual responses. And the oldest children in the forced-choice group even chose mentalistic strategies more often than external ones. Mentalistic strategies are becoming increasingly important to preschoolers. Children have notions of cognitive emotion regulation strategies at a younger age than researchers previously thought.

Another means of regulating emotion is the mere passage of time, which does seem to heal many (if not all!) wounds. Young children are just beginning to understand that the strength of an emotion often changes with its duration (Brown et al., 1991). Brown et al. found that grade school children could describe the unilinear waning of happiness, sadness, or anger at five time points subsequent to an emotion-eliciting event, but that 4- to 6-year-olds were able only to describe change from one emotion to another over time. For these young children, an emotion's diminishment was more difficult to imagine than a concrete transformation of emotions. They also reported that emotional intensity would remain high across time, despite the fact that they could differentiate the high and low emotional intensities inherent in stories (e.g., the happiness of getting a present vs. the happiness of playing records with Mother). Again, preschoolers are just beginning to acquire more complex notions about emotional regulation. The whole idea of time is rather foreign to them, and superimposing it upon another difficult set of concepts, emotion regulation, may just result in "overload."

## Summary

In sum, preschoolers seem to understand that something can be done to regulate emotions; they know a great deal about external strategies, and the oldest preschoolers are picking up mentalistic strategies. They have difficulty dealing with the way emotions can dwindle over time.

## DEVELOPING A KNOWLEDGE OF EMOTION DISPLAY RULES

As stated in Chapter 2, children's expressive patterns become more complex as they grow older; they more often mask, minimize, or substitute one emotion for another. It is important for children to acquire and follow cultural, familial, and personal rules for expression of emotion. But even though there is evidence that young children *use* such rules, very little empirical research has examined preschoolers' *understanding* of dissemblance of emotion and display rules (but see Josephs, 1994).

Although the investigation of preschoolers' knowledge of display rules is just beginning, it is becoming clear that young children recognize situations that call for dissemblance—the act of expressing an emotion that in fact differs from what is felt. This understanding continues to develop through grade school; it is an important element of learning the "feeling rules" of one's culture. Knowing when and when not to show emotions is immeasurably valuable in maintaining social relations, and this knowledge adds to the child's growing emotional competence.

## Dissemblance

The most elementary notion about the reality and appearance of emotion is that of dissemblance. Hiding emotions by masking all emotional expression or substituting one emotion for another can be advantageous to young children as early as they can pose expression voluntarily (see Chapter 2). Dissemblance does not require knowledge of display rules that are normative to a family or culture, but merely the need to send an emotional signal which differing from the one that is felt.

An ingenious investigation of young children's understanding of dissemblance adopted "theory-of-mind" methodologies to assess emotions' reality and appearance, as well as beliefs about them (Gross & Harris, 1988). Children were asked to say how the protagonist in stories *really* felt and *appeared* to feel, as well as how each of two bystanders *believed* the protagonist felt. They heard stories about a protagonist who experienced emotion-eliciting situations. Sometimes this protagonist showed other characters his real feelings; at other times he hid his true feelings, or dissembled. Stories in which the protagonist showed how he really felt were "nondiscrepant" stories, whereas stories where he dissembled were "discrepant" or "deception" stories. All the children understood the *real* feelings of the protagonist in both nondiscrepant and discrepant emotion displays. If the protagonist felt sad about getting an injection or being teased, children demonstrated that they understood what emotion the situation would evoke—even though the protagonist showed his sad feelings about the shot in one story, but in the other story deceived his brother about his sadness about the teasing.

In more complicated, "partially discrepant" stories, one bystander also gave the protagonist a situation-specific reason to dissemble to the other (e.g., "You should not hurt Grandmother's feelings by showing what you feel"). Dissemblance was not inherent in the stories. In these partial discrepant stories, even determining the protagonist's *real* feelings was difficult. The skills of the older children were highlighted: The 5-year-olds were more accurate than the 4-year-olds. Perhaps the younger, more concrete children thought that such an injunction could really change the protagonist's internal state. They may have interpreted the reason to dissemble as "You should not hurt Grandmother's feelings by *feeling that way.*"

In terms of knowing how the protagonist *appeared* to feel ("How does he look on his face?"), nearly all the children gave accurate responses for nondiscrepant emotions; this was expected, given preschoolers' general understanding of emotional situations. But the 5-year-olds were more accurate than the 4-year-olds at telling how the protagonist *appeared* to feel for both types of discrepant emotions, partial and total deception. They understood that where there was any deception at all, the protagonist would *appear* to feel a way different from his true emotions. His face would not show the same emotion he felt. In contrast, younger preschoolers were again more likely to think that appearance could not differ from reality—that "what you feel is what you see." This limitation suggests that younger preschoolers' difficulty in understanding deception is more broadly based in their somewhat less developed theory of mind.

As for beliefs, the children were asked what the bystander thought the protagonist was feeling: "Did David's friends think he was happy, sad, or just okay [when he was really sad but looked happy on his face]?" Children of both ages were more accurate in judging what the bystander believed for nondiscrepant than for discrepant emotion displays. But the 5-year-olds were more accurate than the 4-year-olds in making either judgment.

Inferring others' perceptions of a person's dissembled emotions was admittedly difficult for all young children, over and above judgments of how the person really felt and appeared to feel. Perhaps it was just too difficult to add one more level of inference to the task—to ask a young child to *think* about how another person *thought* about what the protagonist was *trying to project* about what he was *feeling*. Although the 4-year-olds exhibited difficulties in explaining dissemblance, the results of these studies suggested that 5-year-olds' failures to understand dissemblance were not solely due to difficulties in determining a person's real and apparent emotions.

To find out more about such understanding, Banerjee (1997a, 1997b) told 3- to 5-year-olds that the central character in each of six stories about emotions "might really feel one way inside but look a different way on her face. Or she might really feel the same way inside that she looks on her face. I want you to choose the pictures for how she really feels inside, and how she looks on her face" (p. 115) This central character was motivated to hide an emotion, either positive or negative: "Diana wants to hide her brother Bill's toy because he hasn't been very nice. She does so and feels happy, but she needs to hide this happiness so that Bill will not shout at her" (p. 115).

Even 3-year-olds were able to distinguish real and apparent emotions in these situations. Banerjee had implemented several methodological simplifications, compared to Gross and Harris's (1988) study. These included (1) use of pictures to aid the children's responding; (2) fewer questions (i.e., no probes for memory of the story); and (3) explicit statements of how the protagonists really felt, so that the task *only* involved identifying the dissembled emotion. They showed a better understanding of the distinction between appearance and reality for negative, as opposed to positive, emotions. Boys in particular evidenced difficulty conceiving that positive emotions would be dissembled, paralleling the finding that preschoolers have difficulty imagining how to change positive emotions of parents.

So preschoolers, even young ones, have some coherent ideas about the distinction between real and apparent emotion. But, although Gross and Harris's and Banerjee's experimental procedures were intended to reflect common situations in which preschoolers might dissemble, and to make queries simply, they may still have been too taxing, especially for 3- and 4-year-olds. To follow up on the potential underestimation of young preschoolers' understanding, Gross (1993) investigated 3- and 4-year-olds' understanding of both false beliefs and false emotions. Children were asked to determine a puppet's beliefs about a doll with a sad or happy mask, and about felt-tip markers with the wrong color caps. The children, but not the puppet, witnessed the doll putting on a mask to cover its real feelings, as well as the incorrect placement of marker caps (e.g., the blue cap was placed on the red marker). Despite their own privileged information, 4-year-olds and many 3-year-olds understood that the information available to the puppet led it to believe in both a false emotion for the masked doll, and false colors for the markers.

An intense focus on competence–performance issues—where children can show an ability with some methodologies, but not with others—alerts involved adults that this period is a time of emerging skill in understanding dissemblance. Even 3-year-olds can distinguish between emotional experience and expression, and know that a dissembled emotion can create a false belief in another person, when they are given concrete examples of misleading emotional displays rather than stories. Hence, knowledge of dissemblance and deception is beginning to develop in this age range.

But the transition to fuller understanding is not complete until the end of the preschool period. Six-year-olds easily refer to unobservable phenomena, such as motives and intentions, in explaining what a person appears to feel: "She looked like she felt okay, not sad, so that the other children wouldn't laugh and call her a baby." In contrast, 4-year-olds' attention is riveted on observable phenomena, such as the emotional events themselves. They then err by overlooking dissemblance: "She looked sad because they squirted her with the hose." Methods that circumvent this concreteness allow younger preschoolers to discover and acknowledge differing emotional reality and appearance.

## Knowledge of General Display Rules

As noted in Chapter 2, dissemblance is not the only way in which children modify their expressiveness; they also modify their emotional displays to conform to socially or personally appropriate display rules. Although there is not much research on the topic, they may begin to consciously understand such display rules as they begin to use them. After all, they comprehend that objects may really not *be* as they look, know that emotions are personal internal states, and use display rules (Cole, 1986; Wellman & Banerjee, 1991; Wellman & Woolley, 1990; see Chapter 2). Following this line of reasoning, Banerjee (1997a, 1997b) thought that methodological simplifications would unveil preschoolers' true understanding of display rules.

In Banerjee's display rule assessments, a stuffed doll described an emotional experience and asked the child whether or not it should express the emotion. Four of the stories were restrictive; that is, social norms suggested that the emotion be hidden (e.g., Grandma made a "yucky" casserole and the doll wanted to scrunch up his or her face and spit it out, but Grandma was standing right there). The remaining three stories were permissive; that is, social norms allowed emotional expressions (e.g., the doll was happy at Dad's birthday party, and wanted to shout, "Happy birthday!" and give him a big hug). Approximately three-quarters of the preschool-age children responded appropriately to the stories. They knew that emotions should be more often modified in restrictive, rather than permissive, stories. Girls did respond more accurately than boys (see the discussion of girls' *use* of display rules in Chapter 2).

Display rule differences for positive versus negative emotions were examined for restrictive stories: Children responded with "do not show the emotion" more for positive than for negative restrictive stories. For the negative restrictive stories, they advocated truthfully expressing vulnerability. As with dissemblance stories, 3-year-olds gave the fewest appropriate justifications for their answers. Three-year-old girls provided more appropriate justifications than boys, although this pattern was reversed at age 5. Correct justifications most often centered on avoiding negative consequences of displaying true emotions.

Despite my generally sanguine view of young children's developing understanding of dissemblance and display rules, much remains to be done to untangle the levels of complexity that surround these issues. Some reports still suggest that early childhood is a time when these abilities are rudimentary at best (e.g., Gnepp & Hess, 1986). Evidence from this line of research suggests that few children understand, even by first grade, that facial expressions can be minimized, masked, or substituted for prosocial or self-protective reasons. That is, many children do not seem to know—even when their expressive behavior suggests they do—that when a friend wears an ugly sweater, you do not laugh; when your grandma accidentally breaks your toy, you do not show anger; when you lose a contest, you do not cry; and when you steal a cookie, it is best not to look guilty. Despite this assertion, close to half the preschool children in Gnepp and Hess's study cited verbal rules for regulating emotion, such as verbal masking in "I don't care that I lost this silly contest." It is clear that this area remains ripe for convergent results with developmentally appropriate methodologies.

## DEVELOPING A KNOWLEDGE OF SIMULTANEOUS EMOTIONS AND AMBIVALENCE

It is not uncommon for older children and adults to experience "mixed emotions," as when a father is amused at his 2-year-old daughter's antics, but also annoyed with the mess she makes. Because young children's expressiveness is becoming more intricate as they leave the preschool period, they may become conscious of such simultaneous emotions and of ambivalence. They may begin to experience simultaneous emotions and ambivalence themselves, and thus to know more about them.

Several theorists emphasize how difficult it is for children to cite and comprehend situations in which simultaneous but opposite emotions occur. Harter and colleagues propose a cognitive-developmental sequence based on the valence of two felt emotions and the number of targets toward which the two emotions are directed (Harter & Buddin, 1987; Harter & Whitesell, 1989). In this model, children progress through four levels of understanding. The first begins at age 7, when children comprehend that two emotions of the same valence can be directed toward the same target—for example, sadness and anger when a peer wrecks a just-completed puzzle. By age 11, children can acknowledge that feelings of opposite valences can be expressed toward the same target—for example, anger at one's mother for taking away a privilege while loving her all the same. In Harter and colleagues' model, preschoolers' understanding of these emotional issues is embryonic at best.

Yet there is some question whether Harter's group's work underestimates younger children's actual understanding of multiple or conflicting emotions. Again, asking questions via more age-appropriate methodology could reveal that preschoolers have more knowledge than previously supposed. In a downward extension of earlier work (Wintre, Polivy, & Murray, 1990), Wintre and Vallance (1994) investigated 4- to 8-year-olds' abilities to judge the existence, intensity, and valence of multiple emotions. Participants were asked "How would you feel?" after hearing 15 stories, including "For your birthday you get a brand-new bicycle," and "You lose control of your bike and almost crash" (see, e.g., Wintre & Vallance, 1994, pp. 510–511). Children were given the opportunity to rank, on an abacus-like frame, how intensely they would feel happy, sad, angry, scared, and/or loving (depicted pictorially on one axis of the frame). The structure of the task made it easy for children to indicate simultaneity of emotions; instead of their having to spontaneously envision simultaneity, it was almost assumed. Children's most sophisticated responses to the 15 stories were used to categorize their developmental level in judging simultaneous emotions.

Results indicated that at about age 5, children could predict experiencing multiple emotions of the same intensity and same valence to affect-eliciting situations. At about age 6, they began to predict experiencing multiple emotions of the same valence but differing intensities to affect-eliciting situations. It was not until about 8 years of age that children predicted multiple emotions of both varying intensity and opposite valence. Thus, Wintre and Vallance's procedural improvements preserved but accelerated Harter's group's chronology.

Another constructive methodological refinement involves techniques that elicit, rather than spontaneously require, mention of conflicting emotions (Peng, Johnson, Pollock, Glasspool, & Harris, 1992; see also Donaldson & Westerman, 1986). Children heard stories in which a pet or a possession was lost and then found, though in an injured or partially damaged state. This sequence of events would typically evoke both happiness and sadness.

Children were placed in two groups, an "events" group and an "emotions" group. They were then asked two questions about the events in the story. Those in the events group were asked only about events—for example, for the lost-pet story, "Does the child find his pet?" "Is the pet hurt?" In contrast, for the emotions group, the events were assumed. The protagonist's concomitant emotions were elicited: "When the child finds the pet, how does he feel?" "When the child knows that the pet is hurt, how does he feel?"

For both conditions, the third question asked about the child's feelings. For the event group, however, the events were again repeated with only the added question, "How does the child feel?" The children in the emotions group were given two causal statements that linked events and emotions, such as "When the child holds the pet, he is happy that he has found the pet, but he is also sad because the pet is hurt. How does the child feel?" When experimenters highlighted the specific emotions for this group, 6- and 7-year-olds, but not 4- and 5-year-olds, agreed that emotions of different valences were directed at the same target and could explain them. The strategy that involved being told about the simultaneous, mixed emotions across the three questions gave the older group of children the scaffolding they needed to respond correctly. The younger group could not make use of this scaffolding.

In a similar study, kindergartners had much more trouble in *detecting* simultaneous opposite-valence emotions than in *explaining* them (which they could do in 75% of cases; Gordis, Rosen, & Grand, 1989). When these children were told stories similar to "Amir feels happy but also a little sad going to the airport," they were able to explain that Amir was excited to see the airplanes, but felt bad that his father was going on a business trip. In contrast, they could not spontaneously assert that Amir would feel happy and sad at the same time after merely hearing a story describing the same events. Furthermore, when the explaining task was administered prior to the detection task, it highlighted the nature of the task for the children, who then performed better on detecting the simultaneous emotions on their own. In a later study, Brown and Dunn (1996) documented a sex difference in this capability that favored kindergarten-age girls.

These converging results suggest that young children can be sensitive to opposing positive and negative feelings aimed at the same target event. Specifically, preschoolers can recognize and explain conflicting emotions at a younger age than previously reported. In particular, they perceive what it means to have conflicting feelings without spontaneously talking about them. They need priming to discuss these emotional occurrences.

Earlier research also neglected to discern *why* young children have difficulties with mixed emotions. When children are beginning to comprehend so many sophisticated aspects of emotional life, why is this one topic so difficult? Young children's reliance on facial expression to interpret emotions ("Faces can't go up and down at the same time") and on their still-growing theories of mind ("You can't think two ways") gets in their way (Harris, 1983).[1] They may need to "unlearn" some of their most cherished propositions about internal states to move forward in this area of emotion understanding. Highly scaffolded experimental conditions may shed some much-needed light on these issues, by "dissect[ing] the task in order to isolate where problems may occur" (Kestenbaum & Gelman, 1995, p. 446).

Kestenbaum and Gelman set up a series of increasingly scaffolded studies to do just this. In the first, they asked 5-year-olds open-ended questions about feeling happy and sad, happy and angry or sad and angry, at the same time. Sixty-four percent of the children acknowledged that feelings could be mixed. However, their justifications were not especially adequate. Even when their justifications addressed mixed emotions, few children cited simultaneity of feelings or the juncture of two eliciting events. So verbal response demands without any type of support elicited the least understanding about mixed emotions.

Accordingly, the second study required less verbal production. Children heard stories about two distinct but simultaneous events leading to either mixed basic or single basic emotions. Five-year-olds, but not 4-year-olds, were able to discern multiple emotions in the stories, especially when they had visual information. Separation of the emotion-eliciting events made the task easier.

As in weighing expressive and situational aspects of emotion, however, the 4-year-olds' difficulties may have emanated from language and/or cognitive constraints and from lack of experience. Children of this age think more concretely than 5-year-olds; they have trouble with the notion of time and with the linguistic concept "at the same time." Perhaps, too, they have had less experience with the more subtle personal and social experiences that lead to mixed emotions.

In the third, most scaffolded study, these investigators continued their efforts to pinpoint where problems occurred in reasoning about mixed emotions. They capitalized upon and extended the salutary effect of visual stimuli found in the second study. Children were given three types of visual examples of mixed emotions: photographs of adults modified to include the eyes from one emotion and the mouth of another expression; cartoon "aliens" with a similar mix of eye and mouth regions; and cartoon "aliens" with two heads, each expressing a different emotion. Children answered how each stimulus felt in both open-ended and forced-choice formats. In the forced-choice format, 4- and 5-year-olds willingly identified and acknowledged mixed emotions in facial expressions, especially for the two-headed alien; in open-ended questions, they acknowledged mixed emotions *only* for the two-headed alien.

So, given special assistance in visualizing how mixed emotions are experienced and expressed, young children are capable of identifying and talking about them. The methodological addition of the two-headed alien helped the children overcome the disturbing conflict between the existence of mixed emotions and the precept "You can't think/feel two ways."

Despite these encouraging findings, there is still disagreement among developmentalists about whether late-preschool-age children can detect only multiple emotions of the same valence and intensity, differently valenced emotions, or even only sequential emotions directed at the same target (see Peng et al., 1992; Wintre et al., 1990). Nonetheless, preschoolers are beginning to be able to explain conflicting emotions, at least (Gordis et al., 1989). Children's earlier mastery of basic emotion knowledge and their growing skill at talking about the causes of emotions support this budding ability (Brown & Dunn, 1996). As with other areas of preschoolers' emotion understanding, more research initiatives are needed to continue these intriguing lines of investigation. Understanding this element of complexity in their own and others' emotions facilitates a leap in both children's self-awareness and their ability to get along with others. And, knowing that the foundations of this newfound continuity rest in children's individual differences in emotion understanding, parents and caregivers can begin fostering it very early.

## DEVELOPING A KNOWLEDGE OF COMPLEX EMOTIONS

Another big accomplishment in the domain of emotion knowledge is understanding the more complex emotions, particularly the self-conscious and social emotions—guilt, shame, pride, embarrassment, and empathy. Because young children and their peers are beginning to express complex emotions, they have some understanding of them, but it is still emerging. Although they are just beginning to investigate young children's understanding of complex emotions, researchers do know that even the oldest preschoolers are unable to cite pride, guilt, or shame specifically in relevant success, failure, and transgression experiences—pride at a gymnastic feat or resisting temptation, or guilt for stealing a few coins out of the coin jar in the parents' bedroom (Arsenio & Kramer, 1992; Barden, Zelko, Duncan, & Masters, 1980; Harter & Whitesell, 1989; Nunner-Winkler & Sodian, 1988). Children do not use correct emotional terms, or even descriptions, of their own and others' pride or shame until at least age 6. Preschoolers report happiness, gladness, or excitement, rather than pride, for the gymnastic feat. Children even older than this report feeling bad, scared, or worried about detection and the likelihood of punishment after stealing. They do not use terms referring specifically to guilt.

Instead of presenting children with situations and asking how the protagonist would feel, however, Russell and Paris (1994) told children how a story character felt, and then asked them to complete the story by saying why the character felt that way and whether the character felt good or bad. They found that 4- and 5-year-olds have a partial conceptualization of complex emotions such as pride, jealousy, shame, and gratitude: "They understand the [valence] associated with the emotion, but have no knowledge of the kind of situation that evokes it" (p. 349). Furthermore, 4-year-olds through kindergartners usually judge a wrongdoer's feelings on the outcome of his or her actions, using a naive desire-based causal analysis: A person is happy if he or she does not get caught, but angry if caught. They give what has been dubbed the "happy victimizer" response. However, they do not expect a character, even an ill-motivated one, to feel good if he or she harmed another person by accident or observed someone being hurt. Children this young also indicate that they would be sad if they failed at a task. It is important to note that the very nature of wrongdoing realistically elicits mixed emotions, even into adulthood (Murgatroyd & Robinson, 1993). For example, a 5-year-old boy does in fact feel happy that he now "owns" another boy's Power Ranger, even though he stole it from the other boy's cubbyhole. He may also feel scared that he might get caught, or sorry when he sees the other boy crying. But, as noted above, preschoolers' understanding of such mixed and ambivalent emotions is far from perfect. Adding complex moral themes to the mix just makes reasoning all the more difficult.

So preschoolers distinguish between feeling bad and being bad. That distinction is a most basic one, a low-level generalization about the emotional consequences of moral events. Thus, they show that they know emotions are determined not exclusively by goal attainment, but also by limited moral considerations and empathic concern. *Being* bad can actually lead to *feeling* good (and often does!), but witnessing or accidentally causing harm (*being* "good") can lead to *feeling* bad. They also understand the basic breakdown of moral versus nonmoral behavior and feelings, following emotional distinctions that they know best. Basic emotions are, for them, the most logical as outcomes for situations that could elicit the moral emotions of shame and guilt. And overriding concern over wrongdoing does not always "register" in situations where moral issues are central.

Adults who are attuned to children's abilities in this area will be less likely to mismatch their socialization messages to a child's capability to take them in (Arsenio & Lover, 1995). Because the emotional consequences of a sociomoral act are undoubtedly mixed, young children may need adult support to show what they do understand. In studies using probes such as "Could he or she feel another way?" (Arsenio & Kramer, 1992; Lemerise, Scott, Diehl, & Bacher, 1996), even preschoolers could acknowledge feeling both happy and sad feelings after a moral transgression.

Whether they are working from the moral situation to the moral emotion or the moral emotion to the moral situation, preschoolers' understanding is limited to elemental distinctions such as those that supported their earliest understanding of emotional expressions and situations. They still describe the consequences of achievement and moral situations in terms of basic, rather than complex, emotions.

## CHAPTER SUMMARY

Preschoolers' understanding of emotion is not complete, but it is surprisingly acute in a number of domains of emotional experience.

During the preschool years, children become increasingly able to use emotion language to fulfill a variety of functions in their everyday lives. They label emotional expressions and identify emotion-eliciting situations, along with their causes and consequences. Ways of changing their own and others' emotions are becoming clear to them. Finally, they are beginning the long progression toward understanding multiple emotions, ambivalence, and complex emotions such as guilt and shame.

Many situations elicit similar feelings among different people, and facial expressions tend to stand for specific emotions, even cross-culturally. These regularities make it simpler for preschoolers to make inferences about basic emotions; they comprehend situations and facial expressions that are simple and familiar. Children during the period from toddlerhood to late preschool age generally label and recognize happy expressions first, followed by sad, angry, and fearful expressions, in that order. This developmental progression appears in many studies. Receptive recognition often supersedes expressive labeling, as is often the case in language development in general.

Young children also demonstrate considerable knowledge of the causes and consequences of emotional situations. They center on salient qualities of the eliciting situations and of the individuals displaying emotions, whether those persons are themselves, peers, or parents. When these sources of information conflict, children of preschool age are strongly influenced by facial expression in judging emotion, but are beginning to move toward reconciling the two sets of cues. In the absence of an emotional expression, these children tend to infer the emotion that they associate with a situation. The qualities they focus on in inferring causes of emotions fit well within prototype and event structure explanatory approaches.

Preschoolers are also starting to use personalized information to infer how someone is feeling, and sometimes to explain conflicting cues to emotion. That is, when person-specific information readily suggests how that person feels, preschoolers can use this information rather than conflicting normative or situational information. But young children prefer immediately present emotion cues to information about a person's past experience. This preference makes sense, given their limited comprehension of the time course of emotion.

Young children are also aware that emotions may be change-worthy, and are becoming capable of citing effective means of doing so. Although they more often choose behavioral than cognitive strategies to change emotion, preschoolers are capable of generating mentalistic strategies. During the preschool period, children also begin to generate means to change parental emotions, especially their anger. Overall, then, it is clear that notions of both self–other regulation and prosocial reactions to others' emotions are developing.

Methodological intricacies have made it difficult to access young children's comprehension of mixed emotions, display rules, and dissemblance. But when measures are more ecologically valid, preschoolers' nascent abilities in this area are discerned.

Because expressive patterns of guilt, shame, and pride occur later than those of the basic emotions, the lag in understanding of complex emotions or emotions expressed in moral situations is not surprising. More research should be initiated to explore these foundations of children's moral sense, because these social and self-conscious emotions have important ramifications for children's developing abilities to feel good about themselves and to interact with others.

## NOTE

1. This point is probably also true for knowledge of dissemblance and display rules.

# ✿ Chapter 4

# Socialization of Emotional Expressiveness and Understanding

$Y$oung children learn about expressing and comprehending emotions when their parents show emotions, react to their children's emotions, or talk with them about emotions.

*Jamie is screaming at his mother, "I want my snack right now!" "It's too close to dinner time, Jamie. You need to wait," his mother answers as she scrubs carrots at the sink. His eyebrows lower. He glowers ferociously, butts his head against her, and yells again, "Give it now!" His mother remains calm, but sighs deeply. "Jamie, I don't like it when you yell at me like that. In fact, it makes me really sad."*

Jamie's mother unwittingly demonstrates three important ways in which she teaches her son about emotions. First, she models not only calmness in the face of a stressor (Jamie!), but the appropriate facial expression of sadness when verbally attacked by a loved one. Second, she uses developmentally appropriate emotion language. Her speech can assist Jamie in figuring out that some events are often linked with specific emotions: People get angry about not getting what they want, but people also feel sad when they are yelled at. Talking to him as she does also shows him that he can use words as tools, rather than resorting to full-blown tantrums. Third, she reacts to his emotions in a supportive way, while she also suggests the need for regulation.

Many people play important roles in toddlers' and preschoolers' lives—their parents, of course, as well as day care providers and preschool teachers, siblings, and playmates. Information about the nature of emotions and their expression is embedded within even the most minute interactions with others (Denham, 1989, 1993; Denham & Grout, 1992, 1993; Eisenberg & Fabes, 1994; Eisenberg, Fabes, Carlo, & Karbon, 1992; Halberstadt, 1991). In this chapter I describe the key contributions that other people make to young children's growing emotional competence. These other people are called "socializers" because, whether intentionally or not, they show young children what is acceptable in a culture. All of the people who come into contact with a young child are potential socializers of emotions. They can make interesting events happen, have access to things that are attractive, are similar to the child in some way, or are loved by the young child. Of course, parents are the primary socializers, but peers increasingly play a role. However, close contact with parents is important in fostering—or, unfortunately, impeding—the development of emotional competence (see also Goleman, 1995).

Teachers also have varied qualities that make them attractive socializers. They show young children wonderful new skills, direct their play, and form close emotional bonds with them. The emotions that teachers are comfortable sharing give their pupils experience with patterns of expressiveness different from their parents' (Hyson & Lee, 1996). Their reactions to the emotional displays of children in their classrooms can affect how the children cope with their emotions in the future (Denham & Burton, 1996). Whether feelings are discussed openly in the classroom or not also gives important explicit and implicit messages about the world of emotions.

Peers are similar to one another; they can control one another; and they can share enjoyable activities. They are also very attractive to other young children. And of course, anyone who has spent any amount of time in a day care center knows that preschoolers' emotions abound when they come together for play: Friends are often delighted or furious with each other, sometimes hurt each other's feelings, and occasionally get into scary situations. Aptly, more and more peer research is focusing on the role of emotion, and from these reports some evidence can be gleaned. Patterns of expressiveness, for example, are associated with the amount of conflict a child experiences with peers (Arsenio & Lover, 1997). In particular, if a child is often in conflicts and arguments with playmates, the prevalence of the child's negative emotions increases. Frequent exposure to peers' negative emotions contributes to a child's own sadness, anger, and fear through direct imitation, disinhibition, or contagion. In the case of Jamie in the example above, his angry face and "head butt" are very similar to his friend's emotional behavior. Jamie may think anger is okay, or may become angry more easily, after dealing with his friend's ire on the playground all morning.

Older brothers and sisters exert power over their younger siblings, but are also similar to them. Because of these qualities, young children naturally look to them as experts in the feelings business, as in other areas. In particular, those who have closer relationships with older siblings learn much about emotions from them (Dunn, Brown, & Beardsall, 1991; Dunn, Brown, Slomkowski, Tesla, & Youngblade, 1991). The behavior of older siblings guides young children's ideas about what emotions are appropriate for various situations and about how those emotions can be displayed.

Intriguing new research is examining the influence of "other" socializers. Nonetheless, more is known about the parental role. Much of current knowledge about the socialization of emotion rightly (to my mind) focuses on the contribution of parents. So, although many people undoubtedly make powerful contributions to preschoolers' emotional competence, the main focus of this chapter is on parental socialization.

## MECHANISMS OF SOCIALIZATION: MODELING, COACHING, AND CONTINGENCY

Socializers contribute to young children's growing emotional competence—to patterns of expressiveness, understanding of emotions, and emotion regulation (see Chapter 5). Just how do they make these contributions? Three social learning mechanisms have been proposed as processes involved in emotion socialization (Halberstadt, 1991): "modeling," "coaching," and "contingency." These three aspects of socialization—how the socializers show or don't show their own emotions, how they teach or don't teach about emotions, how they react or don't react to the emotions of others, repectively—are key means by which young children absorb the emotional messages of socializers. Maintaining a cheerful demeanor at the pediatrician's office, having a serious chat about a friend who made a child sad, or reacting sympathetically to a tired child's irritable crying are all ways of influencing offspring's expressiveness according to these modes of socialization.

Young children are active social cognizers, always trying to understand what they see, and they pick up on emotional expressions of others as very salient parts of their social world. Modeling of emotional expressiveness happens whenever a parent shows an emotion, and a child observes it; it does not have to be intentional on the part of the socializer. In the following descriptions of mothers' emotion diary entries (see Denham & Grout, 1992), 4-year-olds witnessed the emotional expressiveness of their mothers. It is easy to extrapolate to the impact of these experiences on the children's emotional competence.

*Rachel and her baby sister shared a joyous playtime–coloring, playing with Legos, and singing songs. She saw her mother's happiness and smiled even more.*

*Tyrone learned how anger might be expressed when his mother tried, unsuccessfully, to make a telephone call. She asked him to be quiet and walked into another room, but he followed her and began chasing his sister noisily. She hung up, told him she was very angry, and sent him to his room. He yelled and fussed all the way upstairs. In the same way that Rachel absorbed her mother's happiness, Tyrone took the cues of his mother's lowered brows, her distinctly lowered voice, and her verbal message. He was angry, too.*

*Claire learned about anger and sadness, too. She witnessed an argument between her mother and father. The mother began to cry out of frustration and sadness over the long-standing, unresolvable conflict. Claire watched with eyes wide; she held onto her mother's legs and begged, "Please stop crying, Mommy." Then, getting tearful herself, she said she didn't feel good when her mother cried. Claire went even further than Rachel or Tyrone, using the experience of her mother's sadness and anger in two new ways. She not only became saddened through the contagion of her mother's affect, but added this experience to her knowledge of how sadness is expressed, and also tried to figure out emotion regulation for herself and her mom.*

Similarly, parents' contingent responding to children's emotions fuels emotional competence, or its lack. In the following examples (again based on mothers' emotion diary entries; see Denham & Grout, 1992), parents reacted to 4-year-olds' emotions.

*Jeremy experienced his parents' accepting, helpful reaction to his emotions. He watched the movie Jaws, against his mother's better judgment. He fearfully, animatedly asked many questions about the movie afterwards, and anxiously discussed it in great detail (e.g., "What was that red stuff?") His mother and father answered all the questions and supported him as he resolved these things in his mind. Jeremy's emotions were accepted, and he was able to regulate them, as well as to learn about what makes things "scary."*

*Stacey's mother had bought a new wading pool, and had high hopes for the fun the family could have. But this was a difficult day. Whether told to wait, get in, or get out of the pool, Stacey cried and couldn't be consoled. Nothing could please her. Finally, she had a minitantrum–lying down on the floor, knocking over a chair, and kicking out at things. Her mother told her she couldn't act like that and had to pick up what she had knocked over. She let Stacey cry a while and then consoled her, hugging her and discussing what had happened. Then everyone went back in the pool and had a good time! In this case, Stacey learned that some intensities and means of expressiveness are not acceptable, and that talking about rather than venting feelings can have a positive outcome.*

Finally, parents, some more than others, actively address the world of emotions with their preschoolers, coaching them about it. Here are further examples from the Denham and Grout (1992) study:

*Anikka learned about emotions while looking at a picture book with her mother. A new puppy tried to run away into the path of a school bus:*

MOTHER: *They were frightened. . . . [They] grabbed the dog and brought it to safety. See the worried looks?*

ANIKKA: *They look so scared.*

*Annika learned some new vocabulary for the emotion of fear, new cues for fear, and a new reason to be fearful–the safety of a loved one.*

*Sometimes young children actually initiate clarifying conversations about emotions. Brian's mother felt ill. She told Brian that she could not play because she felt bad. He asked her whether she felt sad or happy. She then told him neither: "I feel sick, not any other way, but I'll be better soon." He hugged her, told her he loved her, and brought her* Sesame Street *magazines to read in bed. Brian learned that sometimes his conjectures about others' feelings could be incorrect, and that the best thing to do is ask!*

With these modes of parental socialization of emotion in mind, many aspects of young children's emotional competence (or incompetence) come into clearer focus. The contributions of their social world are potent and ongoing.

## SOCIALIZATION OF EMOTIONAL EXPRESSIVENESS

In what follows, I first review modeling, coaching, and contingency as means of socializing emotions for a central component of emotional competence—namely, emotional expressiveness. I then review the socialization of more sophisticated expressiveness (i.e., of the self-conscious and social emotions) and of display rule usage. I conclude this part of the chapter with a brief look at how broader socialization experience contributes to expressiveness.

## Modeling Influences on Expressiveness

### Prevalent Emotions

The first way in which parents socialize actual expression of emotion is through their own patterns of emotional expressions, the modeling component. The emotions shown by parents are rich sources of information for young children's own expressiveness. Strong experiences and expressions of emotions are common while parenting preschoolers. When events take place that really matter to parents, emotions follow (Dix, 1991; Patterson, 1980). Things that matter happen all the time; sometimes parents' concerns coincide with their children's needs, and sometimes they decidedly clash. Hence, feelings are ever-present accompaniments to parent–child interactions.

Parents' and preschoolers' concerns and behaviors are often incompatible, leading to negative emotion for parents. A little boy *must* see a certain video *right now*. Siblings squabble, seemingly meaninglessly, over who can carry a certain item of clothing around the house. A parent presses a preschooler to begin complying with demands for simple, familiar tasks. If this child has just thrown rather than put away a toy during the 12th negative interchange of the hour, the parent understandably feels frustrated, impatient, furious, or afraid of his or her inability to teach the child an important lesson. Parental tension and anger are sometimes unavoidable. At the same time, parents' and children's concerns and behaviors can often be compatible, with resultant positive emotions: A mother feels joy as her daughter squeals in delight at climbing a tree by herself. In either case, parental emotions are activated.

Different aspects of young children's expressiveness are influenced by these parental emotions in at least four ways (Barrett & Campos, 1991):

1. Parents unconsciously highlight and discern the emotional significance of events for children. Their expressive patterns implicitly teach the child those emotions that are acceptable in the family and which specific emotions are appropriate for specific types of situations. For example, a 2-year-old girl observes a parent's unease at the approach of a large but friendly dog, and thereafter demonstrates fear herself during similar experiences. She has learned the emotional significance of this situation.

2. Parents model the display of specific emotions and children pick up on these patterns. For instance, particular ways of expressing fear and wariness are conveyed by different parents watching the dog's approach. One parent gasps and exhibits very widened eyes, but another shows much more subtle indicators of wariness.

3. Parents also show children the common behaviors (i.e., "action tendencies"; see Barrett & Campos, 1991) associated with expressions of emotions. They demonstrate their own differing ways of coping with emotional situations, and children of differing parents learn different behaviors for expressing and dealing with emotions. For example, one mother who feels unease at a dog's approach gets up precipitously and whisks the child and herself away from the playground, whereas another, equally wary parent quietly speaks to the dog, assesses risk, and elects to stay at a safe distance.

4. Parents provide an overall affective environment to which the child is exposed. The emotional world view of a child (or of an adult, for that matter) is shaped by the general emotional tone experienced day after day. For example, constant immersion in others' simmering conflicts, or, conversely, typically enjoying others' positive outlooks, has an effect. Eventually the family's emotional milieu puts a unique emotional stamp on a young child's personality. Four patterns of affective environment can be discerned (Tomkins, 1962, 1963, 1991; see also Malatesta, 1990, for an interpretation of Tomkins's work):

a. In the "monopolistic" pattern, a single emotion dominates experience. Parents, for example, may be angry individuals, rarely expressing positive emotions to each other or to their children. A child reared in such a family may be easily annoyed, often cranky, and quick to anger. He or she responds with anger to a variety of stimulus conditions that would not bother other children.

b. In the "intrusion" pattern, a minor element intrudes and displaces a dominant affect. A mother may be quite upbeat most of the time, but may become anxious under specific conditions. For instance, a gossipy sister visits; upon her departure the mother feels jumpy, nervous, and threatened. Her normally cheerful toddler son also adopts this response pattern and reverts to fearfulness and wariness when challenged. A particular child in his playgroup evokes negative emotion.

c. In the third pattern, the "competitive affect" model, the emotion-based aspect of a parent's personality is often in competition with another personality type. Each interprets reality in different ways. One parent "blows up" fiercely, and then is apologetic and placating. The young child then interprets family conflict in terms of anger or misery. Understandably, the child vacillates between sadness and anger in conflict situations.

d. In the fourth pattern, personality styles are "affectively balanced." Parents show a rich emotional expressiveness that gives flavor and zest, as well as information, to their smallest transactions. Here parents are emotionally competent; they understand and can cope with the diverse emotions that arise in social interchange. In these instances, the preschooler experiences and expresses a well-modulated, but not incapacitating, variety of emotions as his or her life experiences warrant.

According to the modeling hypothesis, then, children's expressiveness reflects their parents' own total emotional expressiveness, as well as the particular profile of emotions that the parents express—the prevalence of their happiness, sadness, or anger (Cummings & Cummings, 1988; Denham, 1989, 1993; Halberstadt & Fox, 1990). Children are exposed both passively and interactively to these negative or positive emotions. Either way, they interpret the emotional import of their parents' emotional expression, and tend to express similar profiles of emotions themselves. Indeed, findings reveal that certain expressive patterns of toddlers and their mothers become more and more alike across time (Malatesta et al., 1989).

So, when parents and children interact together, children's emotions are associated with parents'. Positive emotions are contagious: In one study, happier mothers had children who were happier, as well as less sad and angry (Denham, 1989; see also Davies & Cummings, 1995). They enjoyed sharing lunch together, and the children were less agitated when an experimenter assuming the role of a "doctor" asked them to get ready for a checkup.

In contrast, parents' negative emotions are punishing and dysregulating, and this effect is well established by toddlerhood (Davies & Cummings, 1995; Denham, 1989, 1993; Malatesta, 1981). The relations between parent's and children's emotions can be seen easily while they interact. In my study (Denham, 1989), maternal anger and tension were negatively correlated with children's happiness, and anger was positively related to children's sadness and tension. More irritable or more jumpy mothers pushed their children to sit, to eat, to follow instructions; the experience was not pleasant for them, for their children, or even for the observers. So the scaffolding provided by maternal emotions, for better or worse, supported the children's expression of emotions within these situations.

Moreover, the influence of parents' emotions reaches across time and context. Mothers' emotions are related to their children's abilities to cope emotionally during stressful situations when mothers are absent (see Chapter 5; see also Denham, 1989; Denham & Grout, 1992, 1993).

Again, maternal positivity predicts more positive emotion in children. Mothers who showed relatively more happiness during the mealtime and the "doctor's" visit had children who themselves showed more happiness in several situations where their mothers were not present.

Conversely, parents who show negative emotions, especially anger, have children who likewise show less positive and more negative emotions in independent situations. It is more difficult for these children to deal with emotional situations on their own. In the study already mentioned, mothers who exhibited more sadness had children who expressed more anger when the mothers were not present. Maternal anger was associated with children's diminished happiness in the independent situations (Denham, 1989). The contexts experienced without the mothers occurred across several days, suggesting that the effects of mothers' emotions during lunch and the "doctor's" visit were not unique. Rather, they were markers of the general affective environment experienced by the children.[1] Toddlers' emotions when on their own—alone, with another adult, or with a sibling—were reflective of their affective environment.

This contribution of parental expressiveness does not cease as children grow older: Mothers' emotions expressed during interaction with their preschoolers also exert an influence on children's emotions shown during free play in their preschool. In another of our studies, we used interviews and diaries to allow mothers to give their own perceptions both of what emotions they displayed in their preschoolers' presence, and of how they expressed them (Denham & Grout, 1992). As expected, preschoolers whose socialization of emotion was more positive showed more emotional competence with their playmates.

These mothers rated the frequency of various emotions in their daily lives. Those who reported showing not only more frequent happiness, but also less frequent tension, in their children's presence had children who showed more happiness and less anger during free play in the preschool setting. Mothers who endorsed feeling more anger, scorn, and contempt during their everyday lives had children who showed less happiness and more anger in the preschool (Denham & Grout, 1993). Those who expressed negative emotion at home had children who showed more dysregulated emotion during their peer interactions.

Garner, Robertson, and Smith (1997) offer corroborating evidence. In their study, both mothers and fathers reported on their patterns of expressiveness, in general and in their children's presence. Maternal and paternal positive emotions, *expressed around their children,* made unique contributions to their preschoolers' positivity in challenging peer contexts. These investigations add incrementally to the knowl-

edge base about how parental expressiveness socializes child expressiveness. But few have focused on other, more fine-grained aspects of
young children's emotionality. Garner and Power (1996), however,
have found that family positive emotion, as well as sadness, discouragement, and anxiety, predicted how positively children dealt with a
disappointment paradigm.

### Moderators of the Contributions of Parents' Prevalent Emotions

Other ways that parents teach children about expressiveness, over and
above the mere prevalence of their emotions, also emerged as important when we queried mothers via interviews and diaries. Mothers
described important moderators of their expressions, such as the
causes and resolutions of emotional incidents. The *reasons* for mothers'
emotions—the concerns that activated them, to use Dix's (1991) termi-
nology—were crucial to their children's emotional competence in preschool. That is, the effect of maternal emotions differed, depending on
their cause: Children were more emotionally positive when mothers
reported that their anger was not predominantly caused by their
children's disobedience, or that their happiness was caused by their
children (see Denham & Zoller, 1990).

Parents show lots of emotions, and affective environments include
unavoidable tension and anger, especially when preschoolers are key
players! When these negative emotions are strongly felt, their *resolution*
is important (see also Cummings, Simpson, & Wilson, 1993; El-Sheikh,
Cummings, & Reiter, 1996). When mothers apologized to children for
their moments of tension, the children were happier in preschool
(Denham & Grout, 1992). Apologies include comforting emotion
language that allows children to maintain a sunny outlook. Parents
need to tell even young children, "I am very grumpy, but not because
of you. And I'm sorry if I am making you miserable, too." Cummings
and colleagues' work also supports the importance of resolved anger;
even relatively subtle resolutions are associated with children's lessened
distress.

In contrast, when mothers considered their anger *helpful* in child
rearing and did *not* apologize for it, children were more emotionally
positive in preschool. These mothers were citing their sometimes
justified sternness in child rearing: "I am displeased with your behavior." In short, the context of a parent's emotion, not only the emotion
per se, is important in the socialization of preschool emotional competence.

The intensity of mothers' negative emotions also contributed to
their child's sadness. These preschoolers were sadder during free play

when their mothers reported higher-intensity tension, and when they reported crying to express sadness in the children's presence. Such children were immersed in negative emotion and its contagion, and were also probably learning quite specific modes of negative expression.

Moderating influences on the contribution of parental emotion to children's expressiveness often exist in combination as well. In yet another study, mothers were asked to simulate anger while they and their children examined photographs of infants showing emotions (Denham, Renwick-DeBardi, & Hewes, 1994). Unexpectedly, mothers who simulated higher-intensity anger had children who showed *less* sadness and anger during free play in their preschool classrooms. Perhaps these children of high-anger mothers responded with inhibition and lessened emotional expressiveness; or, more likely, mothers of more reactive children may down-regulate their own expressiveness to protect them from anger (see also Fabes et al., 1994). Mothers' and children's overall levels of emotionality undoubtedly interact in their influence on emotional competence shown in the preschool environment.

Alternatively, it may be important to determine the relation between frequency and intensity of each parental emotion, since these two parameters of emotion can interact in contributing to young children's emotional competence. If a negative relation between intensity of anger and its frequency were specified, for example, these findings could be better explained. Perhaps near-constant exposure to lower-level anger is more detrimental than exposure to occasional outbursts of intense anger.

Other combinations of moderating factors need to be uncovered in order to understand the contribution of parental expressiveness to young children's expressed emotions. For example, in the Denham and Grout (1992) study, mothers who said that their anger was frequent and caused by their children's disobedience, and who reported not apologizing for this anger, had children who were sadder when in preschool; the frequency, cause, and resolution of maternal emotion acted in concert. And the unexpected finding in the Denham, Renwick-DeBardi, and Hewes (1994) study might be better explained in the context of the mothers' *reason* for showing higher- or lower-intensity anger during a simulation.

Sex differences in the power of parental modeling as a socialization technique have also been discovered (Denham, Mitchell-Copeland, Strandberg, Auerbach, & Blair, 1997). Specifically, mothers' and fathers' relative balance of happiness over anger predicted daughters', but not sons', positivity in their preschool classroom. Parents' more internalizing emotions—their sadness and tension/fear—were also negatively associated with daughters', but not sons', positivity. Daughters' sensitivity to parental socialization of emotional expressiveness is both a blessing and a curse. The greater salience of the socialization context for girls' behavior needs to be studied more explicitly in the realm of emotional competence.

## Summary

In short, a number of studies provide converging evidence that parents' expressed emotions exert an influence that extends beyond the immediate interactional setting. Children learn about the emotional significance of events—enjoyable, "together times," as opposed to strange, stressful, or conflictual situations. They also learn how to show emotion, both expressively and behaviorally. Above all, they are exposed to an ethos, an affective environment, that has far-reaching effects on the emotional organization of their personalities.

Because emotion researchers study the frequency or duration of parents' emotions most often, most research has so far focused mainly on the contribution of what Tomkins would call monopolistic affect. Results show the child behaviors associated with the predominance of a particular parental emotion. But it is methodologically feasible to identify clusters of parents who show either intrusive or competitive emotional organization—parents who are mostly happy but sometimes fearful, or often angry or sad. These analyses should be undertaken. Nonetheless, the conclusions reached from the current state of research should give caregivers and parents pause. As they become aware of the effects of their own expressiveness, important adults in young children's lives can adjust their own expressiveness for the preschoolers' benefit.

## Coaching Influences on Expressiveness

"The preverbal child is at the mercy of rages and anxieties. . . . This is why the mother and father are at the center of the young child's sense of well-being or despair: they are the ones in charge of understanding the child's experience and attending to it, and they are also the ones who find a substitute to act for them when they are not there" (Lieberman, 1993, p. 47). One such "substitute" is emotion language. Talking about emotions gives the child a tool to use in modulating the expression of emotions (Bretherton et al., 1986; Dunn et al., 1987; Dunn & Munn, 1985; Greif, Alvarez, & Tone, 1984; Kopp, 1989). Parents who talk about emotions and foster this ability in their children enable their children to express certain optimal patterns of emotions, and to separate impulse and behavior.

### Functions of Emotion Language

Emotion language has three special functions in the socialization of emotional expressiveness (Miller & Sperry, 1988):

1. It allows specificity in communicating how to feel, what to say, and what to do in certain situations.
2. It has the "capability of representing the non-here-and-now" (Miller & Sperry, 1988, p. 220), so that socializers can assist the child by reminiscing about emotional experience, anticipating it, and visualizing affective possibilities.
3. Linguistic features, such as the unmitigated imperative to signal anger (e.g., "Get out of here right now!") and intonation (e.g., gruff, clipped speech), allow for a richness of affective communication.

Miller and Sperry's (1987) observations illustrated many of these functions of emotion language within a very specific context. Working-class mothers of toddler girls were observed extensively and interviewed about how they dealt with their daughters' anger. Mothers in this community anticipated the experience of their own and their daughters' anger. According to them, anger needs to be justified by reference to its instigator's actions. Thus, they taught this principle to their daughters via their emotion language: "She sassed me, so I just smacked her," "Jen ran her bike into her, and I screamed, 'Let Jen have it.'" The clear message in this particular setting was that anger is not only okay; it is necessary when one feels victimized.

The way mothers in this study used the language of emotion also provided their toddlers with subculturally important distinctions between legitimate and nonlegitimate anger. What is appropriate to feel, and how should one act to express that emotion, in this particular community? Nonlegitimate anger included acting "spoiled," showing anger merely as a function of frustration. Daughters were pressed by their mothers to act appropriately in emotionally charged situations, and not to "waste" their anger over "wimpy," nonlegitimate concerns.

Young as they were, these girls were even able to give their emotions legitimacy by generating false accusations to justify their expressions of anger if necessary: "She broke my toy" (when she had not). Even finer distinctions were made. Angry, aggressive retaliation was more easily legitimized toward peers than toward adults: "It's okay that she kicked her friend, but she'd better not try that with me. I'm her *mother.*" Differential encouragement of emotions also occurred. Sadness was much less often seen than anger in situations of intentional injury and transgression. People who had been wrong did not get sad; they got even.

The little girls absorbed these discussions and messages, and their patterns of expression were affected by the coaching of their socializers. Although this study makes it clear that not all communities promote the same emotional messages—many middle-class families are less positively disposed toward anger—the principles used by these mothers are very common. Coaching about emotions supports a child's initiation into a social group.

Other research reveals how emotion language helps young children learn how to express emotions. In one set of studies (Denham & Auerbach, 1995; Denham et al., 1992), mothers and their children looked at and discussed photographs of infants showing peak discrete emotion expressions (from Izard et al., 1980). When the mothers considered their conversations complete, they looked back at the photos of the sad and angry babies, and enacted these emotions themselves. The frequency, function, and accuracy of the emotion language used by each dyad member were coded. Functions of emotion language included (1) commenting ("She has a surprised look on her face"), (2) questioning ("She's happy, isn't she?"), (3) explaining ("He's mad because he doesn't like nobody to touch him"), (4) moralizing ("It makes me sad to see [the baby] sad"), and (5) guiding behavior ("I'm gonna be angry if you do that . . . ").

Maternal and child language, especially during the simulations, was strongly correlated with children's emotions expressed in preschool. Some aspects of talking about emotions with mothers were associated with happier, less angry, and less sad experiences in the preschool classroom; mothers who explained their emotions in the simulations had children who were less sad in the preschool, for example. In contrast, mothers who talked on and on about their own distress during the simulations, but without explaining it, had children who looked more affectively *negative* in the classroom. These mothers "wallowed" in negative emotion via their language, conveying a negative emotional style. Their unrelenting, but equally unilluminating, harping on negative emotions was debilitating to the children.

But perhaps neither talking about emotions in a general way while looking at the baby photographs, nor talking about emotions while supposedly experiencing them during the simulations, is the best setting for learning about emotional expressiveness via coaching. Maybe children gain an optimal understanding of their own expressive patterns, and their parents', while reminiscing about emotional events.

Reminiscing about emotions experienced together is a special way of reflecting about strong feelings and ways they can be regulated, in a realistic but calm atmosphere.

In a second set of studies, my colleagues and I focused on such parent–child reminiscences about emotions. Naturalistic conversations were recorded in which parents and children reminisced about their own emotions (happy, sad, angry, and afraid; Denham, Mitchell-Copeland, Strandberg, & Highsmith, 1994; Denham, Mitchell-Copeland, et al., 1997). Mothers who talked more about emotions during these conversations had children who were happier and less angry during free play in their preschool classrooms.

*Summary*

Emotion language is important because it is a means of direct teaching and learning about emotion. This information given young children about emotions can be associated with their own patterns of expressiveness. Often the relation between parental emotion language and child expressiveness is moderated by the specific function served by the emotion language, but it seems clear that maternal talk about emotions imparts important messages about how to show feelings and how to regulate them. Less is known so far about the contribution of fathers' emotion language. Parents and caregivers need to carefully consider open, though not overwhelming, discussions of feelings with their children.

## Contingency Influences on Expressiveness

Others' reactions to children's emotions can be important vehicles for letting children know what action tendencies are appropriate when they feel different ways, and what events merit emotion expression at all. According to the contingency hypothesis (Halberstadt, 1991), parents' own expressed emotions and behaviors are likely to be contingent on their young children's emotion displays (Malatesta & Haviland, 1982). Specific reactions to children's emotions can either encourage or discourage certain enduring patterns of expressiveness in the children themselves, as well as children's mobilization of emotional resources in social situations where they are "on their own."

> *If Kelsey is terrified of entering the swimming pool–crying, eyes wide, feet pushing back from the side of the pool–her somewhat embarrassed, goal-oriented, but loving parents could act in at least two different ways. They could ignore her fear, saying something like "Oh, Kelsey, stop it, this*

*will be fun, let's just try it! Splash!" Alternatively, they could respect the intensity of her feelings and sit down with her near the pool, saying, "I would never let anything hurt you." And if she were unable to calm down, these parents would give up on this new experience for that day, or maybe the foreseeable future.*

The second reaction would help Kelsey become less fearful in other situations, first with her parents present and later on her own (Malatesta, 1990; Tomkins, 1991). Her fears need not monopolize, or even unnecessarily intrude upon, her emotional experiences. They will undoubtedly be experienced and expressed, but can be modulated and dealt with. Hence, two types of reactions to children's emotions—rewarding and punishing—shape their emotional responses to particular eliciting situations, and ultimately contribute to the emotional organization of their personalities (Tomkins, 1991).

Usually we think of parents as socialization agents, with good cause. But peers can also participate in this type of emotion socialization. Peers' immaturity often leads them in the direction of punitive socialization; in peer situations, one's anger is often responded to in kind (Denham, 1986) and with escalated conflict. The social costs of such anger also include rejection by the peer group (Arsenio & Lover, 1997; Denham & McKinley, 1993; Denham, McKinley, Couchoud, & Holt, 1990; Lemerise & Dodge, 1993). Children are likely to be gleaning unique socialization messages from their peers!

## Rewarding Contingency: Contributions to Children's Expressiveness

An affectively balanced, "integrated" emotional organization is fostered when caregivers exhibit primarily rewarding reactions—when they assist the child in maintaining positive affect, and tolerate the child's negative affect as valid and worthy of regard and concern rather than disgrace.

*Three-year-old Monroe feels very sad because his very first best friend has to move away. His rewarding parents help him say goodbye, allowing him to experience the sadness, but also to know the value of relationships. They suggest ways to manage the sadness, such as "writing" letters. They freely reminisce about this good friend and about good times shared, telling Monroe that this good feeling can happen again. They assist him in moving through his sadness, rather than criticizing it.*

Overall, Monroe's sensitive parents assist him in enacting strategies that reduce negative affect, subsequent to its usefulness as a social signal. They focus on helping him to cope with this source of affect and to avoid unnecessary irritation. Above all, they remain affectively engaged with him while he experiences negative affect. They communicate this attunement facially and verbally, nurturing his sympathetic affect and action by their example.

Rewarding parents take their children's emotions seriously. "Listening attentively, asking questions to clarify what the child believes, and offering a reassuring explanation as well as the promise of protection," as well as "remain[ing] emotionally available even while firm" (Lieberman, 1993, pp. 35 and 39), constitute the core of successful socialization of emotion. Rewarding socializers do "much to help their children with each of the basics of emotional intelligence [or competence]: learning how to recognize, manage, and harness their feelings, empathizing, and handling the feelings that arise in their relationships" (Goleman, 1995, p. 191).

### Punishing Contingency: Contributions to Children's Expressiveness

Punitive socialization leads to far less positive developmental outcomes. Punitive socializers are "dismissers" of emotion (Gottman, Katz, & Hooven, 1996a, 1996b). Some dismissers want to be helpful, but ignore or deny their children's emotional experience—treating emotions as something to blow over, or even a trivial bother. They "fail to use emotional moments as a chance to get closer to the child or to help the child learn lessons in emotional competence" (Goleman, 1995, p. 191).

*Rebecca is afraid of the dark. Punitive socializers are likely either to ignore her, to focus on their own needs, or to distract her, so that she never really deals with the experience. In any case, she is still left with the fear.*

Or dismissers may be just too *laissez-faire*; they may okay any alternative a child selects to handle emotions, or resort to distraction even when other means of coping are possible. All upsets are soothed, and even bargaining and bribery are used to stanch the flow of negative emotions.

*Brandon's parents allow him to show his continuing anger about being picked on at school, but they are exhausted by the whole topic. When the anger floods him, he screams at his mother, "I am angry at you! I hate you!" They distract him with ice cream for dessert, offering no means of regulation or pressure to express emotions in a more useful way.*

In a final, most pernicious way, dismissers may be full of contempt, showing no respect for how the child feels. "They might, for instance,

forbid any display of the child's anger at all, and become punitive at
the least sign of irritability" (Goleman, 1995, p. 191).

*Scott's parents, who are punitive socializers, show disregard and even
contempt when his best friend moves away. These parents tease Scott for
his tender feelings, so that in the end he is let down not only by the
disappearance of his friend, but by their reaction as well. Unlike Monroe,
he is very lonely and still feels very bad.*

### Parents' Reports of Their Contingent Reactions to Preschoolers' Emotions

Some investigators gather parents' own self-reports about their reactions to children's emotional expressiveness (e.g., Casey & Fuller, 1994;
Casey, Fuller, & Johll, 1993; Eisenberg & Fabes, 1994; Eisenberg, Fabes,
Schaller, Carlo, & Miller, 1991). Parents give eloquent testimony about
their own reactions to their children's emotions. They describe how
they deal with their children's emotional responses in common emotion-provoking situations, and mention their own specific emotions
directed at their children (e.g., Casey et al., 1993).

Invariably, though, the picture is not so simple as "be a rewarding
socializer, raise super kids." The ability to be rewarding socializers is
related to parents' predominant form of expressiveness, as well as to
how parents feel about their children. Parents who themselves are more
emotionally positive in general are more capable of being rewarding
socializers of emotion for their young children; those who depict their
families as positively expressive are more accepting of their children's
emotional responses, and more likely to cite verbal reassurance as a
strategy they would use to help their children regulate emotion (Casey
et al., 1993). Conversely, parents who describe their families as less
positively expressive focus more on altering their children's emotional
responses, are less accepting, and propose more active intervention
strategies aimed at suppressing or changing their children's emotions.
Feeling "bad" themselves leaves little emotional room for parents to be
rewarding socializers. And parents in more negative families probably
need to exert pressure on their youngsters to down-regulate their
emotionality.

The contingent responding reported by parents is also related to
how they feel about their children. Those parents who describe their
children as enjoyable and easy to deal with are more accepting of their
children's negative emotions. In contrast, parents who tend to feel
anger toward their children are less accepting and expect conformity
to parental expectations. These parents are also less satisfied with the
children's responses. Their ability to accept and foster their children's

emotional experience, and their need to control it, are rooted in the very nature of their affective relationship with their children.

Consonant with this emphasis on relationship, it must be underscored that parents' contingent responding is related to their children's own enduring emotional expressiveness—in other words, to their children's temperament. Children's effects upon their own socialization of emotion must not be overlooked; emotional development is very transactional in nature. Hence, it is not surprising that mothers report they are distressed by and try to minimize, children's expressiveness, especially when the children are viewed as high in negative affect, emotionally intense, or low in attentional control (Eisenberg & Fabes, 1994). Some children pose a challenge to parental equilibrium, and thus are pressed to regulate themselves. Similarly, it is easier to encourage expression of emotion and emotional problem solving when children themselves are able to focus and switch their attention easily. Thus, although in this discussion much of the onus is placed on the rewarding or punishing qualities of parents as socializing agents, children play an active role in the very nature of their socialization experiences.

### Observation of Contingent Reactions to Preschoolers' Emotions

Parents' reports of their own contingent reactions to children's emotions have yielded important insights. Another way of gleaning information on the contingency hypothesis is to *observe* parents' specific emotional and behavioral reactions to children's emotions (e.g., Casey et al., 1993; Casey & Fuller, 1994; Denham, 1993; Denham & Grout, 1993; Denham, Renwick-Bardi, & Hughes, 1994; Denham, Mitchell-Copeland, et al., 1994, 1997; Malatesta et al., 1989). Maternal punishing reactions to toddlers' emotions predicted the children's own emotions (Malatesta et al., 1989). Toddlers' sadness during reunions within the Strange Situation was predicted not only by the their own sadness in similar situations when younger, but also by their mothers' earlier lack of interest (these effects were moderated by child sex and birth status). Likewise, children's anger during reunions was predicted not only by their own earlier anger, but also by mothers' surprise at their earlier sadness. So there was not only cross-time stability in toddlers' expressiveness, but also prediction of later expressiveness from mothers' earlier contingent reactions. When mothers were not rewarding socializers of emotion, toddlers continued to demonstrate negative emotion.

Mothers who responded optimally to their toddlers' happiness, sadness, anger, and fear also had children who coped better with their own emotions when the mothers were absent (Denham, 1993). Specifically, maternal positive responsiveness to child sadness, anger, and fear during mealtime and the "doctor's" visit predicted children's happiness, fear, anger, and affiliation when mothers were not present, even after the effects of child age and gender, and of children's own patterns of emotional expressiveness with mothers, were accounted for (Denham, 1993).

What are reasonable reactions to young children's emotions? Optimal reactions to sadness include behaving with tenderness and not showing negative or happy responses. Appropriate reactions to angry displays include displaying calm neutrality or cheerfulness and not matching a child's anger. Angry responses only lead to continued angry, noncompliant behavior on the child's part (Crockenberg, 1985). Optimal responsiveness to a child's fear include calmness, cheerful caretaking, or modeling of appropriate, nonfearful problem-solving behavior. Nonoptimal reactions include responding with anger, sadness, tension, or overplacating tenderness, which only serve to prolong the child's distress. Even smiling that occurs too soon after a child's happy display can be nervous or "fake" and can overstimulate a young child (Malatesta et al., 1989). In sum, an emotionally available parent assists a child in tolerating, confronting, and managing negative emotions, rather than minimizing them at all costs.

Parents' emotional reactions to their preschoolers' emotions are also related to these older children's expression of emotions (Denham & Grout, 1993; Denham, Mitchell-Copeland, et al., 1994). Parents who are emotion "coaches" in this way foster their preschool children's emotional competence on a variety of indices (Denham, Renwick-DeBardi, & Hewes, 1994). In sum, these rewarding socialization techniques promote the integrated emotional organization of personality.

## Moderators of Contingency

*Age of Child.* Although it is reasonable to expect both age and sex differences in socialization via contingent responsiveness, little empirical evidence exists. Age differences have, however, been found in both well and depressed mothers' reactions to their young preschoolers' anger (Kochanska, 1987). Mothers of young children in the sample, from 15 to about 30 months of age, were more likely than mothers of children from 30 to 42 months old to provide affection, gratification, or distraction, and to inquire about the cause of the anger. In acknowledgment of growing expectations of their children's increasing autonomy and self-regulation, mothers of older children were more likely to suggest cognitive strategies to their children, and to ask them to stop displaying anger.

There are also age-related differences in the consequences of these socialization techniques. Parental matching of their children's positive emotions predicted children's prevalence of happiness over anger, but more so for 4- and 5-year-olds than for 3-year-olds (Denham, Mitchell-Copeland, et al., 1997). Older children were more able to use this positive matching as an actual template for their own expressiveness. As Grusec and Goodnow (1994) have pointed out, the effect of parental socialization is dependent upon the children's own perception, understanding, and acceptance of the message!

*Gender of Parent and of Child.* The study by Casey et al. (1993) pointed to important differences, as well as similarities, between the socialization of emotion of mothers and fathers. Mothers were more realistic than fathers in admitting that children's emotions in response to an emotional situation would not necessarily match their own wishes. Mothers were also more likely than fathers to say they could modulate their children's emotions. Mothers' greater day-to-day experience with preschoolers made them more realistic about the volatile nature of their charges, and the need to regulate their capricious expressiveness. Of interest was the finding that fathers did not differ from mothers in their empathy for and acceptance of children's feelings. Fathers also unexpectedly exhibited a range of ways to assist children during emotional experiences—as diverse as mothers'.

Casey et al. (1993) also found that parents socialized the emotions of boys differently from those of girls. They wanted boys to inhibit sad and fearful responses, whereas girls were expected to inhibit angry responses. These expectations fit well with cultural norms: "Big boys don't cry," "Girls make nice."

Sex differences in the potency of contingent responsiveness as a predictor of emotional competence occur as well. Parents' antisocial reactions to children's emotions (e.g., yelling, making the situation worse) predicted daughters', but not sons', sadness and fear in the preschool classroom (Denham, Mitchell-Copeland, et al., 1997). Furthermore, Kochanska (1987) found that well mothers were more attentive to and concerned about their sons' anger than their daughters' (see the parallel finding on coaching of emotion understanding, below). They more often offered angry boys affection, gratification of their perceived needs, and cognitive strategies. This pattern was reversed for depressed mothers and their young daughters, perhaps because of the dependent, role-reversed nature of their relationships; depressed mothers wanted to maintain their helpers' equilibrium.

Again, child sex is an important moderator of the socialization of emotion, and it needs to be more fully explored.

## Summary

Caregivers want to help their children experience a well-modulated, rich emotional life that enhances rather than incapacitates. It is vital that they carefully consider the impact of their contingent responses to their children's emotions, and oversee the emotional interchanges between peers, without "smothering" their spontaneity.

## Socialization of More Sophisticated Expressiveness: Self-Conscious and Social Emotions

Most exploration of socialization of emotional expressiveness is new enough that it still focuses on young children's expression of basic emotions. But a few investigators are beginning to examine the foundations of more advanced milestones in the development of expressiveness, such as the self-conscious and social emotions. With the exception of the socialization of children's empathy, this research often does not directly map onto the rubric of modeling, coaching, and contingency influences, however. This state of affairs is not surprising, given that the complexity of the self-conscious and social emotions rests on more deliberately made cognitive distinctions than those for the basic emotions. In the following accounts, I convey current information about the socialization of three of young children's complex emotions: shame, guilt, and empathy.

### Shame and Guilt

*Shame.* Often the "moral" emotions—shame and guilt—are engendered by socialization that includes an amalgam of modeling, coaching, and/or contingent responding, along with attributions about the child's worth, culpability, responsibility, or care for others. In the case of shame, the mechanisms of socialization of emotion posited here are coupled with other sorts of messages that pervasively degrade the child.

*A habitually overtaxed and exhausted mother, after spending several hours with her perpetually whiny, fidgeting preschooler, Denise, finally snaps: She states venomously, "You are such an idiot!" She has acted angry, but she has also given Denise clear and damaging information about her worth. The next day, when Denise plays quietly with a new game for an extended period, the mother says nothing.*

Once children have learned standards and rules for behavior, parental reactions like these can engender shame (Lewis, 1992). Denise knows that she has done a bad thing by her very existence, and she feels shame.[2] There is no socialization of emotion technique at play in the second episode, but neither is there any approbation for achievement and good behavior.

Self-reported shame in 5- to 12-year-olds is more clearly related to parents' expression of emotion—specifically, to "absence of [positive] discipline, the strong presence of *hostile emotion*, little recognition of good behavior . . . [and] little in the way of concrete feedback regarding what the child had done that was right or wrong" (Ferguson & Stegge, 1995, p. 190; emphasis added). As for children's expression of other negative emotions, the strong presence of anger figures prominently in the development of shame, especially in the absence of positive parenting (see also Moskowitz, 1997). In parental shame induction, the anger is often accompanied by disgust, as well as by disciplinary techniques of love withdrawal and humiliation.

Whether conveyed by modeling, coaching, or contingency mechanisms, such affective messages are extremely dysregulating to young children. They lead to another important aspect of the socialization of the experience and expression of shame—the children's internalization of negative attributions about their own ability and worth, as implicit in the example above (see also Zahn-Waxler & Kochanska, 1990, although they do no distinguish guilt and shame as sharply as Tangney et al., 1995, or Ferguson & Stegge, 1995). In such a context of socialization of emotion, a child's experience of shame seems almost overdetermined.

More details on these attributional contributions to the experience and expression of shame were uncovered by Alessandri and Lewis (1993). Parent–child interactions were videotaped during easy and difficult puzzle, copying, and basketball-toss activities. Parents' verbalizations were coded as global or specific regarding their content ("You are a good ballplayer" vs. "You placed that piece just right!"), and as positive versus negative with respect to their affective tone. Thus, each verbalization fell into one of four cross-classified categories. Children whose parents made specific negative evaluations about them expressed more shame across all three activities, of both difficulties, with both parents. When parents made positive specific or global statements, children evidenced less shame. Girls received fewer of these positive specific evaluations, and more of the specific negative ones, suggesting a reason for them to become more shame-prone than boys.

*Guilt.* Both shame and guilt emerge after the child internalizes standards for behavior. Guilt, as specified in Chapter 2, is more closely allied with misbehavior than shame, which is related to deficiencies in the self. Ferguson and Stegge (1995) searched for the roots of guilt, along with shame, in young children. In contrast to shame, guilt was associated with parents' blame and anger after misdeeds and failures, and with their pride in positive encounters. Children who demonstrated guilt had parents who said that they had done a bad *thing* that caused displeasure, rather than that the children *themselves* were bad. When parents reported a higher discrepancy between their children's actual behavior and what it ought to be, but a lower discrepancy between their children's actual self-regulation ability and what it ought to be, there was also more guilt. This constellation of parental correlates paints a picture of a child who is seen as able to self-regulate and behave well, but who does not do so in a particular morally important encounter: "You could have left the vase on the table. You didn't have to knock it over. But you did. I'm so disappointed in your behavior." The parents' communication of this view contributes, according to Ferguson and Stegge, to the child's feeling naughty or sorry after a transgression.

*Summary: Guilt and Shame.* In sum, caregivers' actions are related to their children's emotions of guilt and shame; in particular, their negative emotions that are strongly expressed together with personally evaluative statements or behaviors are linked to shame. More parents and teachers need to know this, because they would not want to induce shame if they understood its pervasive negative effects. Even though a modicum of guilt probably motivates amending behavior, parents and teachers should carefully consider socialization practices contributing to either guilt or shame. Parent education programs should be fine-tuned to include a focus on rewarding and punishing socialization of emotion, particularly spotlighting the problems inherent in shame induction. Along with safeguarding against the promotion of guilt and shame, however, parents and teachers also want to foster empathy—the sympathetic concern for others that motivates prosocial behavior.

## Empathy

Although the experience of empathy—feeling the same emotion as another person is experiencing—can engender personal distress, it often includes sympathetic concern (see Chapter 2). This sympathy facilitates social interactions; children who spontaneously help playmates are viewed positively by them (Eisenberg, Pasternack, Cameron, & Tryon, 1984). How are such emotional responses to the predicament of other people promoted?

Many aspects of parental expressiveness are central to the development of sympathy. When children have experience with clear but not overpowering parental emotions, they have the opportunity for empathic involvement with others' emotions. They are more likely to evidence concern, and to help, comply, commiserate with, or cheer up their partner—instead of becoming upset, just watching, or doing nothing at all.

Revisiting studies mentioned earlier, with an eye to the expression of sympathy and sympathetic behaviors, is useful here. Specifically, mothers' prevalence of negative emotions during either laboratory play sessions or home visits, especially anger, negatively predicts children's prosocial responsiveness to peer emotions during free play in their preschool classrooms (Denham & Grout, 1993; Denham, Mitchell-Copeland, et al., 1994; Denham, Renwick-DeBardi, & Hewes, 1994). In contrast, mothers' more affectively balanced emotional expressiveness (i.e., more positive than negative emotions) is a positive predictor of these empathic reactions. Negative emotions shown in an overall positive context allow for the development of sympathy. More consistent exposure to parents' negative emotions is painful for young children and generally impedes the development of sympathy.

Other qualitative aspects of parents' emotional expressiveness around their children are central to both the development of general expressiveness (see Chapter 2) and the development of empathic responding. Intensity of maternal negative emotions, and the presence of concurrent unresolved conflict, are also associated with less mature patterns of responses to peer emotions: less help and concern, but more frequent sustained attention. Hence, not only the specific emotions shown by parents, but their intensity and the resolution of negativity, are important in inducing children to experience empathy and behave sympathetically.

Furthermore, children in the Denham and Grout (1992) study were most prosocially responsive to their classmates' emotions when mothers said they (1) explained their sadness; (2) expressed their tension more positively when it affected their children; or (3) expressed their relatively infrequent anger rationally to their children. Positive, rational means of knowing why and how their parents feel emotion are most productive in inspiring children's empathy. This makes sense, given the sympathy–personal distress dichotomy. Such parental socialization provokes other-oriented sympathy, as opposed to self-focused personal distress:

*Madeline's mother is sick and tired of her daughter's dawdling. As the mother feels her temper rising and hears her voice becoming sharper, she*

*stops and takes a deep breath so her anger does not intensify. The "fit"*
*she feels coming on would do no one any good. She sits down beside her*
*still-playing daughter–it is time for school–and sternly says, "Maddie, I*
*am getting really frustrated. You must put on your shoes." Later in the*
*car, she reflects, "You know, I'm glad we got that settled. You were really*
*a good helper when I told you what we needed." The mother has expressed*
*her anger rationally, and Madeline will be more empathic with others'*
*frustrations in the future. She knows that others' negative emotions have*
*reasons and can be resolved.*

Parents' contingent responsiveness to emotions is also important
in the socialization of empathic responsiveness. What do parents do
when their children are distressed or anxious, or show socially inappropriate emotions? Do they exhibit anxiety or sympathy themselves?
How do their reactions map onto their children's reactions to peers'
distress (Eisenberg et al., 1992, 1993)?

It makes sense that children who live in a sympathetic environment
learn to follow suit. Children who observe optimal emotional and
behavioral reactions to their own and others' emotions have templates
to follow in empathic involvement with peers (Zahn-Waxler, Radke-
Yarrow, & King, 1979). When mothers show certain benevolent patterns of reactions to others' negative emotions, children show less
egoistic distress and more sympathetic concern to the distress of others
(Fabes, Eisenberg, & Miller, 1990; Eisenberg et al., 1992), as well as
more prosocial behavioral reactions to the emotion displays of peers
(Denham, 1993; Denham & Grout, 1993).

In a series of studies on these questions by Eisenberg et al. (1992,
1993), there were also a number of significant relations between
parental self-reports about socialization of emotion and their reports
of their young daughters' responses to others' distress. When mothers
and fathers reported that they would try to downplay the girl's
expressions of emotions that would hurt others, such as contempt, they
saw their daughters as exhibiting less helping and comforting toward
distressed peers. This parental pressure to restrict certain emotions
was, however, related to daughters' emotional sympathy unaccompa-
nied by assistance. Because of their parents' socialization, these young
daughters experienced a strong empathic reaction internally, but were
reluctant to enact the behavioral action tendency associated with their
empathy on behalf of a distressed peer. They considered *all* emotions
as needing to be hidden.

These results, taken together, suggest that exposure to parents'
regulated and nonoverwhelming displeasure gives young children practice in prosocial responsiveness within the parent–child relationship,
which then generalizes to the peer setting. More long-lasting, intense
negative parental emotions, unexplained and unresolved, so distress

young children that the process of induction is short-circuited through the pain of guilt, information overload, or incapacitating fearfulness. Rewarding contingent responsiveness also gives children a guide to follow in reacting to others' emotions.

## Socialization of Display Rule Usage

Given the unfolding story of socializers' contribution to children's expressiveness, it follows that parents are also likely to convey information about when and when not to display emotional expressions. Wrinkled brow, compressed lips, and lip biting are expressive patterns that suggest dampened negative emotion. Parents' use of these patterns is associated both concurrently and predictively with toddlers' early use of the same display rules, suppressing negativity to fit cultural expectations (Malatesta et al., 1989).

The parental emotions experienced by preschoolers during interaction and in the more general affective environment also contribute to their ability to perform according to emotional display rules. Mothers' self-reports of internalizing negative emotion in their families were related to children's inability to show positive expressions after a disappointment, even when the effects of children's own emotional intensity and emotion knowledge were controlled for (Cole, Zahn-Waxler, & Smith, 1994). Children who lived in a sadder, more internalizing, more muted affective environment were less able to "put on a good face" when disappointed.

In contrast, when mothers themselves maintained a positive demeanor when their child received a disappointing gift, their children were less likely to show negative expressions during the disappointment. Children whose mothers tempered the disappointment by "cheering them up" were less likely to behave in a negatively expressive, impolite manner toward the experimenter. The sparse research available, then, suggests that at least the modeling aspect of socialization of emotions is important to young children's developing use of display rules. Little or nothing is known yet about the contribution of parental coaching and contingent responsiveness to young children's display rule usage. This area is ripe for investigation.

## Broader Socialization Experience Contributing to Expressiveness

Other aspects of children's social interactions and relations with socializers, over and above those directly related to emotions, are important contributors to the development of emotionally competent expressiveness. Nonetheless, there is little research supporting this proposition, with the exception of some promising work on attachment and empathy.

The attachment relationship plays an important role in the development of emotional expressiveness, particularly of empathy (Zahn-Waxler & Radke-Yarrow, 1990). The interplay of cooperation and turn taking, and, above all, positive affect sharing and distress relief—all hallmarks of a secure attachment—would be especially vital in this regard (Kestenbaum, Farber, & Sroufe, 1989; Thompson, 1990). In fact, the attainment of a secure attachment relationship with a caregiver can be seen as a precursor to the aspects of emotional competence discussed here. I will return to this theme in Chapter 7.

In the Kestenbaum, Farber, and Sroufe (1989) study, groups of 4-year-olds, equally distributed across secure, anxious–avoidant, and anxious–resistant attachment statuses, were observed during play. Empathy-evoking instances where at least one child was visibly or audibly distressed, and one or more other children were near enough to be able to witness it, or someone else responded from a distance, were sought. Every child who witnessed the display was rated on "empathy" and "antiempathy" scales incorporating both affective and behavioral information. Experience in a supportive relationship contributed to these youngsters' empathic sensitivity: Children who had been classified as secure during infancy scored higher on empathy than children with anxious–avoidant histories. Moreover, 9 of the 12 incidents of antiempathy, in which one child actually exacerbated another's distress, involved children with avoidant histories as exacerbators.

Early relationships are prototypes for later ones, with expectations within early relationships carried forward to new ones (Sroufe & Fleeson, 1986). The secure children in this study, then, replicated the sensitive caregiving that they themselves received in times of distress. In contrast, the children with avoidant attachment histories did not experience emotional availability in the same way; accustomed to avoiding emotions in their early relationships, they continued to do so by not responding or responding inappropriately to peers' emotions.

## Summary: Socialization of Emotional Expressiveness

Overall, there is much accumulating evidence pointing to various elements of parents' and other caregivers' modeling, coaching, and contingency contributions to the expressiveness patterns seen in young children. The emotions we adults demonstrate, the ways we talk about emotions, and the ways we react to children's emotional experiences are important contributors to children's enduring patterns of emotional expressiveness. More research to flesh out the patterns of parental socialization more fully—via not only parents' monopolistic emotional organization, but also their intrusive or competitive expressive profiles—and even more articulated views of rewarding and punishing socialization are necessary. Furthermore, fuller views of the moderating influences of child age and sex, and of fathers' special contributions, are needed. More work also needs to be done on the socialization of more complex emotions and display rule usage. In addition, I would like to see what lies behind all the correlational evidence that is accumulating. If maternal positivity predicts child positivity, for example, what actual cognitive, emotional, and social *processes* are at work to account for the association? Experimental paradigms such as those discussed by Cummings (1995b) could be used advantageously.

Finally, the scanty research available suggests that researchers should also look at other aspects of social interaction, especially interaction with peers and siblings, to unearth contributors to emotional expressiveness. It is clear that both peers and siblings exert modeling, coaching, and contingency influences on preschoolers' emotional expressiveness.

## SOCIALIZATION OF UNDERSTANDING OF EMOTIONS

Aspects of socialization also contribute to individual differences in young children's understanding of emotions. Parents' talking about emotion-laden experiences in daily life, their encouragement of emotional expression in children, and their own expression of predominantly positive emotions all promote children's emotion knowledge (Denham, Zoller, & Couchoud, 1994). A body of evidence on the contribution of overall positive parenting techniques to children's emotion understanding also exists.

### Modeling Influences on the Understanding of Emotions

*Contributions of Modeling to Understanding Expressions,*
*Situations, and Causes of Emotions*

Parents' expression of emotions can teach children specifically about emotions. Conversely, parental expressiveness can make it more difficult to address issues of emotion altogether. By modeling various emotions, moderately expressive parents give children information about the nature of happiness, sadness, anger, and fear—their expression, their probable eliciting situations, and their more personalized causes. For example, when his mother claps delightedly upon opening the mail, a preschool boy sees that receiving a long-awaited package calls for an expression of joy.

Exposure to well-modulated negative emotion is related to understanding of emotion. In families where there is some conflict and negative emotion, children will "have opportunities to observe models and gain instruction about the appropriate ways to express negative affect" (Garner, Jones, & Miner, 1994, p. 624; see also Widlansky, 1994).

> *Mother's tears when Aunt Joan calls to tell her of their father's (Rashida's grandfather's) grave illness show Rashida one cause for sadness and one way to express it. As Daddy pats Mother's hand and strokes her back, the linkage between sadness and care is also reinforced in Rashida's mind. Later, Mother and Daddy are sharing the drive to Grandfather's. As they approach a bridge that goes up, up, up, Mother licks her lips and her eyes dart from side to side. She does not cry out, but Rachel knows she is afraid. Rashida and her older brother—though he rolls his eyes and sighs audibly in mock disgust—see not only that even big people can be scared, but also that they have learned ways to minimize their expressiveness.*

Recent research upholds these notions. When mothers reported somewhat negative feelings about their children, their children verbally enumerated more causes for sadness; they were well versed at feeling sad themselves (Denham & Zoller, 1990). Bowling and Jones (1993) found that maternal subordinant negative expressiveness, such as sadness, predicted kindergartners' knowledge of emotional expression, even when children's age and receptive language ability were statistically controlled for. So a moderate degree of experience with at least the more internalizing negative emotions can contribute to emotion knowledge.

But when parental emotions are more frequent, intense, and negative, children are disturbed and dysregulated (Crockenberg, 1985; Denham & Grout, 1992; Hoffman, 1984; Parke, Cassidy, Burks, Carson, & Boyum, 1992). When this occurs, the children experience heightened personal distress during emotionally charged events; this self-focus diverts attention away from facial and situational information about emotion, so that little is learned. If, instead of being charmingly expressive, Rashida's mother were constantly "blowing her top" in extreme, intense, hurtful ways, Rashida's knowledge of emotions would probably be restricted. Likewise, little information about emotional expressions and situations is imparted by parents whose expressiveness is quite limited.

My colleagues and I have conducted several studies to evaluate the contributions of socialization predictors to children's understanding of emotion (Denham et al., 1992; Denham, Zoller, & Couchoud, 1994; Denham, Renwick-DeBardi, & Hewes, 1994). Regarding maternal expressiveness, mothers' emotions were coded second by second during an approximately 90-minute laboratory playroom visit. Furthermore, as mentioned above, mothers' means of simulating sadness and anger during a structured task were categorized as either highly emotional with predominantly empathic and guilt induction, or less emotional, with a more intellectualized approach to conveying the emotion to the child.

Maternal emotional expressiveness predicted children's emotion understanding. Moreover, these studies again highlighted the power of maternal anger as a *dis*organizer of social-emotional development (see Cummings, Iannotti, & Zahn-Waxler, 1985; Cummings, Zahn-Waxler, & Radke-Yarrow, 1981; Denham, 1989; Dunn & Brown, 1994): Maternal anger expressed during interaction with the child was negatively correlated with emotion understanding. The mothers of children low and high in emotion understanding differed in amount of anger displayed. "Stars" of emotion understanding had mothers who were lower in anger; the mothers of less adept children showed more anger. Children of mothers who experience higher levels of anger directed at their children are specifically less able to demonstrate comprehension of angry situations (Garner, Jones, & Miner, 1994). Maternal tension and sadness also are often modestly negatively associated with various separate indices of emotion understanding. It is easy to imagine the confusion and pain of young children who are relentlessly exposed to their parents' negative emotions. It is no wonder their emotion understanding is compromised.

## Contributions of Modeling to Understanding of Display Rule Usage

Very little work has been done on parental emotions' specific contributions to more advanced levels of preschoolers' emotion understanding, such as understanding of display rule usage. Preschoolers' and kindergartners' knowledge of display rules—in situations such as losing a game, seeing someone in silly pajamas, not liking a present, or watching a parent leave on a trip—was associated with mothers' self-reported emotional expressiveness, even after children's age and receptive language ability were statistically controlled for (Bowling & Jones, 1993; Jones, Abbey, & Cumberland, in press). First, knowledge of self-protective display rules was related to maternal dominant negative emotions, such as anger and contempt. When children knew that their mothers could react intensely, even explosively, they also knew ways to "cover up" emotions to avoid trouble (e.g., covering up their guilt after stealing a cookie). Less happy mothers might also require their children to be more in control of their expressiveness (e.g., not laughing in church). Their children's uncontrolled emotionality was the "last straw" for these dysphoric mothers. In contrast, prosocial display rules were negatively predicted by maternal subordinant negative expressiveness, such as sadness. Sad, morose, emotionally self-focused mothers were less able to convey to children how expressiveness can be managed for the sake of kindness (e.g., not showing disgust at Grandma's casserole).

### Summary

In general, then, exposure to negative maternal emotions, especially anger, often impedes the process by which children come to understand emotion. The role of less externalizing maternal emotions, such as sadness, is less clear. Some exposure to these more internalizing emotions can be beneficial to the development of emotion knowledge. Knowing that adult emotions are pivotal to the accumulation of one more core emotional skill may motivate parents and caregivers to be more conscious of their socialization influences.

## Coaching Influences on Understanding of Emotions

According to the coaching hypothesis, parents encourage children's exploration and understanding of emotions directly. They verbally communicate to children the experiential meaning of emotions (Saarni, 1987). Such communication heightens children's awareness of emotion within parent–child interaction, and motivates them to attend to and process such emotional information.

> While looking at a photograph of an intensely sad, crying infant, one mother in our studies (Denham et al., 1992; Denham, Renwick-DeBardi, & Hewes, 1994) had this exchange with her 3-year-old daughter:
>
> MOTHER: Have you ever felt like that? You know what I'd feel like if I were like that? I'd feel like nobody likes me at all. . . . What would you do if I was feeling like that?
>
> ASHLEY: I would ask Daddy if he could hug you.
>
> MOTHER: Give me the kind of hug you would give me. . . . Poor little [baby]. Oh, he must feel so bad. That's a real big sad. He looks like his little heart is broken.
>
> Ashley's attention was riveted on the conversation, on the photograph of "Jason," and on her mother's face.

Obviously, such parent-led conversations about the names, causes, and consequences of different emotions specifically aid the child in his or her active attempts to link expressions, situations, and words into coherent, predictable schemas about emotional experience (Bullock & Russell, 1986).

## Family Conversations about Emotions

In short, these conversations about emotions further the child's developing social cognition of emotions (Brown & Dunn, 1991). As these authors asserted, "Discourse about the social world may in part mediate the key conceptual advances reflected in . . . social cognition" (p. 252).

Naturally occurring conversations about feelings between mothers and their 18- to 36-month-old children show how maternal emotion language teaches children about feelings (Brown & Dunn, 1991, 1992; Dunn et al., 1987; Dunn & Munn, 1985). By the time toddlers reach 18 months, mothers and children discuss the causes of emotions, particularly the toddlers' own. From 24 to 36 months, mothers change their feeling state language to parallel their children's usage (see Chapter 3): They refer more often to others' thoughts, feelings, and desires, and their use of emotion language to control behavior ("Stop crying," "Now calm down") decreases.

Individual differences in mothers' usage of emotion language and its various functions teach children to use emotion language in specific ways. When viewing photographs of infants showing emotions, the emotion language of both mothers and their children was embedded in discourse that fulfilled a variety of functions, such as commenting, questioning, explaining, attempting to change another's behavior, and moralizing (i.e., a "little sermon"; Denham et al., 1992; see also Bretherton et al., 1986). Mothers especially used more questioning and explaining than their children, commensurate with their role as teachers; however, there was no mother–child difference in the use of emotion language to guide behavior ("You're making me sad"). Young children already know how to use emotion language to influence others!

Family talk about emotions is transactional; the issues brought up by one conversation partner are tackled by the other. Children who talked to their mothers about feelings had mothers who also talked to them about feelings at both 33 and 47 months (Brown & Dunn, 1992). Children's emotion language directed at siblings was predicted by siblings' emotion language as well. So, when the other member of a dyad uses emotion language, even a young preschooler is more likely to do so as well.

Examination of the function of each partner's emotion language helps to elucidate this pattern even further. In the Denham et al. (1992) study, cross-correlations between children's and mothers' emotion language were not marked by a simple pattern of "I talk more, you talk more." Rather, when mothers asked more questions about emotions, children answered by using more emotion words in explanations. When mothers explained emotions, their children asked fewer questions and used less frequent guiding language, suggesting that they were more satisfied with complete information. Children's guiding language was correlated with mothers' use of guiding emotion utterances. More accurate mothers also had children who used more accurate language—that is, who described emotions more appropriately.

In general, mother–child talk is complementary; a mother tends to talk about the child's own emotions. In contrast, child–sibling conversations about feelings tend to be reciprocal, with each dyad member manifesting his or her own emotional point of view. This distinction is important. Coupled with recent evidence that preschoolers talk more about emotions with siblings and friends than with mothers (Brown, Donelan-McCall, & Dunn, 1996), a transition can be seen from the foundation of "emotion language with mother" to the even more mature, social-competence-enhancing "emotion language with equals." Hence the particular relationship between persons talking about emotion makes a difference in the content of preschoolers' feeling state conversations. Children learn about distinctive aspects of emotion from different conversation partners.

But does mothers' emotion language at one point in time predict children's emotion language later? Is more going on than children's being able to carry on a conversation contemporaneously, as admirable as that may be? Will they be able to use emotion language more ably later if their mothers use it with them? New evidence reveals that mothers who use a lot of emotion language at one point in the preschool period are not doing so simply because their children are also doing so: When mothers and older siblings discuss emotions with toddlers at 18 months, their children also talk more about emotions at 24 months (Dunn et al., 1987). Preschoolers whose mothers used more emotion language in parent–child conversations about past emotions at one point in time used more emotion language themselves later in time; the contrasting child-to-mother effect did not exist (Adams, Kuebli, Boyle, & Fivush, 1995; Fivush, 1989; Kuebli, Butler, & Fivush, 1995; Kuebli & Fivush, 1992, 1996).

*Contributions of Coaching (via Emotion Language) to Understanding*
*Expressions, Situations, and Causes of Emotions*

Associations between maternal emotion language and children's broader
emotion knowledge also appear later during preschool. Both total emotion language usage and specific function usage predict children's concurrent and later understanding of emotion (Denham et al., 1992;
Denham, Zoller, et al., 1994; Dunn & Brown, 1994; Dunn, Brown, &
Beardsall, 1991; Dunn, Brown, Slomkowski, et al., 1991). Dunn, Brown,
Slomkowski, and colleagues (1991) examined the connection between
mother–child emotion language at 33 months and understanding of
emotion at 40 months. Both child-to-mother and mother-to-child feeling
state talk, especially a child's talk about causes of emotions, were related
to the child's understanding of emotion as assessed by my puppet
measure. Similarly, feeling state talk at 36 months—again, both child-to-
mother and mother-to-child—was related to the child's later understanding of emotions at 6 years (Dunn, Brown, & Beardsall, 1991).
Importantly, none of these associations were moderated by the children's
verbal fluency or general linguistic experience; the specific importance
of emotion language in the family is underscored.

   We too found that mother–child emotion discourse is important
in predicting children's ability to identify emotion expressions and
situations (Denham et al., 1992). The accuracy of children's emotion
language with mothers was related to their scores on our puppet
measures of emotional expression identification and situation comprehension. The accuracy of their mothers' emotion language was also
related to the children's ability to label emotional expressions. Mothers
who repeated children's emotion language during the photograph
discussion had children who displayed greater knowledge of emotion
situations. In addition, mothers who talked more about the emotions
they simulated, using more comments and explanations, had children
with greater emotion knowledge overall (see also Garner, Jones, Gaddy,
& Rennie, 1997).

   Those mothers who spontaneously explained their emotions during the laboratory simulation had children who were more adept at
understanding emotions (see also Dunn, Brown, & Beardsall, 1991;
Dunn, Brown, Slomkowski, et al., 1991). Their highlighting of personally relevant emotion information by repeating the children's utterances or explaining their own feelings (e.g., "You make me sad when
you don't sit still") aroused their children and captured their attention.
Guilt-tinged, quickly processed, salient "hot" cognitions ensued in the
children (see Hoffman, 1984). Such cognitions, resulting from this

inductive style of discipline, are fertile ground for the social-cognitive development of emotion understanding (Hoffman, 1975; Hoffman & Saltzstein, 1967; Maccoby & Martin, 1983).

Research evidence from at least two major laboratories indicates that feeling state conversations between mother and child contribute to the preschooler's growing causal reasoning about the common situations in which emotions occur. Verbal give-and-take about emotional experience within the scaffolded context of chatting with a parent helps the young child gradually formulate a coherent body of knowledge about emotions' expressions, situations, and causes.

Such personally relevant discourse about emotions centers on young children's and their parents' own experiences of negative emotion (Dunn & Brown, 1994). This affective context is a special window of opportunity for young children to learn about the causes and consequences of emotions. Unfortunately, however, less talk about feelings occurs when young children are experiencing emotion and family negativity is high. Perhaps the negative relation between maternal anger and children's emotion understanding, then, is due not only to the children's oversensitization to emotion, but also to the disinclination of mothers experiencing negative emotion to talk about emotion themselves. Children likewise process personally relevant emotion information best when they are calm. So reminiscing about emotional experiences, even after a relatively brief time delay, is a beneficial tactic (see also Chapter 6).

## Gender as a Moderator of Coaching's Contribution to Understanding of Emotions

Are there gender differences in this socialization via coaching? In general, parents and older siblings talk more about emotions to preschool-age girls than to boys (Dunn et al., 1987; Fivush, 1989; Greif et al., 1984; Kuebli & Fivush, 1992, 1996). By 24 months, girls themselves referred to feeling states more often than did boys. In North American culture, females are assumed to be more emotional and more interested in emotion; these results, although not replicated in all studies, fit with such assumptions.

Even the type of emotion and the contexts of emotion deemed appropriate to discuss are exposed to gender-related pressures. To pursue this line of argument, Fivush and colleagues also explored ways in which mothers and their 30- to 70-month-old children discussed emotional aspects of their past experiences; mothers not only directed more total feeling language and more unique emotion words to girls, but also discussed anger much more often with sons and sadness more often with daughters (Fivush, 1989; Kuebli et al., 1995; Kuebli & Fivush, 1992, 1996). Moreover, they placed emotions in an interactional framework to a much greater extent with daughters. These differences began to show up in children's own emotion language. By 3 years of age, girls were using substantially more emotion language, with the difference increasing across the preschool years. Differences in the ways girls and boys discuss emotions with others can influence how they come to think about their emotional lives over time (Kuebli & Fivush, 1992). Girls think of emotions as something to share with others, whereas boys learn to express anger directly, but not to talk about it to others as much.

*Summary*

In short, coaching works as a means to increase emotion knowledge. Caregivers should be encouraged at the growing body of information on this aspect of emotional competence. Clearly, there are some moderating factors involving the type of emotion language used, its function, the way it is imparted, and the sex of the child to whom it is imparted. Nonetheless, the major finding is that talking about emotions with young children is beneficial to their development. We need to know more about fathers', teachers', and siblings' contributions to this development, however.[3]

# Contingency Influences on Understanding of Emotion

According to the contingency hypothesis, parents' emotional and behavioral reactions to their children's emotions also help the children in differentiating among emotions. Again, rewarding socialization of emotion is associated with the most positive child outcomes. Children of parents who encourage emotional expression have more access to their own emotions than do the children of parents who value maintenance of a more stoic, unemotional mien, and thus come to understand emotions better.

> *Jonathan can speak about subtle differentiations in his own anger at the bully in his class. Partly he is just plain mad, and wants to punch Donald; partly he is mad only a little, because he doesn't know why Donald hates him. His parents listen, and when he is angry they validate his feelings, letting him know that it is okay to feel this way.*

But they very easily could dismiss the irritable torrent of "Donald this" and "Donald that" that emanates from Jonathan at the dinner table.

Thus, parents' varying reactions to the child's expressions of specific emotions also suggest to the child those situations when they are and are not appropriate. Jonathan is learning more than when to express emotions; he is learning about the very nature of emotions themselves.

### Rewarding Contingency: Contribution to Children's Understanding of Emotions

Mothers' emotionally positive responsiveness to children's observed emotions predicted preschoolers' emotion understanding in one study (Denham, Zoller, & Couchoud, 1994). Positive responsiveness included reacting with happiness to children's happiness, with tenderness to their sadness, and with calmness to their anger. So mothers who were more tolerant and positive (i.e., who conformed more closely to the rewarding socialization prototype) had children who were able to identify emotional expressions and situations, even those requiring some personalized inference. For example, Claire's mother (see "Mechanisms of Socialization: Modeling, Coaching, and Contingency," above) was tolerant of Claire's distress during the argument between the parents; she talked to Claire calmly and tenderly as she tucked her into bed. Her approach to Claire's emotional experience was consistently responsive in this manner. When questioned about her knowledge of emotions, Claire was able to see the viewpoint of the puppet who felt differently than she did: "Well, I really like to go swimming. But he is really, really scared, so I will put the scared face on him."

### Punishing Contingency: Contributions to Children's Understanding of Emotions

As expected, mothers' *lack* of emotionally negative responsiveness predicted preschoolers' emotion understanding in this study (Denham, Zoller, & Couchoud, 1994). Negative responsiveness included reacting with anger to children's sadness or anger, or with happiness to their sadness. One pattern of responsiveness initiated escalating cycles of negativity; the other constituted "making fun" of a child.

Parental behaviors contingent on children's emotional displays also influence their understanding of situations that elicit emotions; we focused on these in our next series of studies. Either negative reinforcement or ignoring of a child's emotions by mother *and* father was a negative predictor of emotion understanding (Denham, Mitchell-Copeland, et al., 1994, 1997). Negative reinforcement was generally indexed by directly or indirectly telling the child to stop showing an emotion—for example, by distracting the child. The contributions of such negative reinforcement were significant even after we statistically controlled for the contribution of intrapersonal contributors, such as age, gender, children's own reactions to parental emotions, and cognitive/language ability. Hence, parents showing behaviors that fit the punitive socialization paradigm had children who were less adept at age-appropriate emotion knowledge tasks.

Mothers' self-reports about their own negative reinforcement in emotion socialization were also revealing. Those who reported that they discouraged their children's emotional expressiveness ("I think children must learn early not to cry," "I do not allow my child to get angry with me") had children who were less adept at comprehending angry situations, or even broader measures of emotion knowledge (Denham & Zoller, 1990; Garner, Jones, & Miner, 1994).

## Age and Gender as Moderators of Contingency's Contribution to Children's Understanding of Emotions

Child sex, however, moderated the contribution of the parental responsiveness to child emotion: Maternal negative emotional responsiveness was a negative predictor of boys', not girls', emotion understanding (Denham, Zoller, & Couchoud, 1994). Because girls obtain more coaching about emotion than boys, sons may rely more on more indirect mechanisms of contingent responsiveness to acquire emotion knowledge. In this way, boys are especially vulnerable to such punitive socialization.

Age of the child was also found to be an important moderator of socialization effects. In particular, younger children who experienced negative reinforcement following their emotional displays showed less advanced understanding of emotion (Denham, Mitchell-Copeland, et al., 1997). Younger preschoolers especially need to be open to their own experience of emotion in order to begin comprehending more complex emotions. We found that their willingness to consider emotional events and issues was especially stymied by this dismissing approach. Older children's emotion knowledge, on the other hand, benefited more from parents' matching of their positive emotions. Younger children are most affected by the contagion of such reactions, whereas older ones are more able to discern such behaviors as distinctive reactions to their own particular emotions, fueling their emotion knowledge.

## Summary

Despite the complexity of the overall story, there is support for key ideas about how children learn about emotion. Rewarding socialization practices allow preschoolers to experience many expressive patterns, and to reflect on even negative emotions, thus promoting their emotion understanding. Across several studies and ways of depicting responsiveness, effects of contingent responses to children's emotions were found to be consonant with notions about rewarding and punitive socialization of emotion.

## Overall "Positive Parenting" Influences on Understanding of Emotions

At the most molar level, components of generally positive parenting contribute to emotion understanding. At least two groups of researchers have addressed this molar level (Abraham, Kuehl, & Christopherson, 1983; Denham, 1996b). Maternal and paternal limit setting and reasoning, as well as maternal intimacy with the child, were related—though in complex, age-dependent ways—to young children's understanding of emotional expressions and situations (Abraham et al., 1983). Mothers' use of reason to help children learn acceptable behavior was related to emotion knowledge, regardless of child age (Abraham et al., 1983; Denham, 1996b). In fact, mothers who resorted to guilt induction in their reasoning, actually appealing to their children's affective connection to others in order to gain compliance, had children who spontaneously verbalized more causes of emotion (Denham, 1996b). Paternal reasoning guidance was related to younger, but not older, preschoolers' understanding of emotion (Abraham et al., 1983).

Paternal limit setting—including consistency of setting and enforcing limits, and the extent to which daily routines were defined—was negatively related to younger preschoolers' understanding of emotion. Similarly, maternal limit setting was negatively related to older preschoolers' understanding of emotion (Abraham et al., 1983). I also found (Denham, 1996b) that mothers' inconsistent limit setting was positively related to children's understanding of emotional expressions and situations,[4] as well as to accuracy of emotion language when examining infant emotion photographs, across two samples. In contrast, indulgent mothers (those who were not necessarily inconsistently applying limits, but just not applying them at all) had children who demonstrated less understanding of emotional situations, particularly ones requiring somewhat personalized inferences.

How can these results be explained? Parents who value order and rules may be less apt to address the world of emotion. Families where disciplinary rules are less consistently followed may be more relaxed and open to both positive and negative emotional experiences, from which the children learn. Alternatively, when limit setting is inconsistent, children may need to become attuned to parental affect by necessity: "Is Mother angry now, and does she 'mean business' this time?" In contrast, where there are few rules at all, there is little pressure to learn about social relations at all, including the emotional domain.

When mothers endorsed free expression of emotion—indicating willingness to let their children observe and/or hear their own emotions, including fear, annoyance, and frustration, and to let them observe their disagreements with other people—younger preschoolers demonstrated greater understanding of emotion in Abraham et al.'s study, as well as identification of emotional expressions in my research. Seeing maternal emotions exposes children to circumstances where emotional expressions and situations can become clarified.

In contrast, maternal intimacy—mothers' openness in expression of physical affection to the children and others in the children's presence—was negatively related to younger preschoolers' understanding of emotion situations. As with limit setting, emphasis on this aspect of parent–child relations, which is admittedly positive in an overall sense, precludes more direct tutelage about emotions. Perhaps in this case, intimacy is associated with a more overprotective shielding from emotions.

Parents who self-report using most positive parenting techniques, then, create an affective environment in which emotions are openly shown and discussed. As such, the home is a crucible for learning about emotions' expressions, situations, and causes. It is revealing, however, that some parenting techniques are generally positive for child development overall, but not quite as beneficial for the development of this specific component of emotional competence. Furthermore, the age-specific and sometimes parent-specific associations of parenting techniques and emotion knowledge underscore the complexity of the picture.

## Other Factors That Contribute to Understanding of Emotions

### Peers and Siblings

Interacting with other children is another important aspect of social experience that promotes the development of emotion understanding. A central tenet of Piagetian notions about affect and intelligence is that socializing with others at one's level of development, where negotiation and renegotiation are necessary, brings the young child to a new level of awareness. For example, Jonathan's best friend is probably less patient than his parents about putting up with Jonathan's grousing about Donald. He tells Jonathan, "Be quiet!", and Jonathan learns more about the nuances of emotion—specifically, that complaining and fussing can stimulate answering annoyance.

Unfortunately, very little research has focused on the socializing influence of peers and siblings. But, consonant with these theoretical premises, practice and experience in bouts of pretend play at 33 months (especially with siblings) was related to emotion knowledge at 40 months (Youngblade & Dunn, 1995). It is easy to imagine pretense, where one child acts the role of the crying baby and another responds as the comforting mother, as a stage on which a panoply of emotions are acted out. The participants feed each other's emotion knowledge. Intriguingly, more emotional children also engaged in more pretend play, which then stimulated their emotion knowledge. More positive mother–child and sibling–child relationships were also associated with a greater amount of pretend play. Children's growing emotion understanding, then, is grounded in their own emotionality and their own relationships: pretending, deceiving, teaching, joking, comforting (Dunn, 1988, 1995).

Older siblings are particularly potent socializers of emotion knowledge, because their relationship with their younger brothers and sisters is characterized by power amidst egalitarianism and love amidst conflict. A colleague has recently uncovered tantalizing indicators of this richness (Sawyer, 1996): When older siblings show a rewarding socialization pattern, reacting positively to positive emotion and not ignoring either positive or negative emotion, their younger siblings demonstrate more proficient emotion knowledge. Similarly, cooperative interaction with older siblings is associated with preschoolers' contemporaneous use of more sophisticated emotion language, and with their later ability to comprehend ambivalence (Brown et al., 1996; Brown & Dunn, 1996).

### Self

As potent as socializing agents' influence can be on young children's developing emotional competence, there are also child effects on each of the phenomena. These child effects include age as a marker for cognitive development, linguistic development, and other, unspecified developmental change. Parents, researchers, and caregivers alike need to recognize that despite preschoolers' formidable abilities in emotional competence, there are some intrapersonal limiting factors. Thus, before expecting certain levels of understanding of emotion or particular expressive patterns, a caregiver would be wise to consider each individual child's age, as well as his or her levels of cognitive/linguistic ability and development of self. Moreover, elements of emotional competence itself are interrelated: A child who is more emotionally expressive may have more experiences to fuel his or her understanding.

## CHAPTER SUMMARY AND CALL FOR CONTINUED PROGRESS

Developmental psychology is still in the early years of studying the socialization of preschoolers' emotional competence, but already much has been learned. Parents' modeling, coaching, and contingent responsiveness contribute to children's enduring emotional expressiveness, as well as to their ability to comprehend basic emotional expressions and situations. Other important contributors to emotional competence, such as cognitive development and the attachment relationship, are also beginning to be uncovered. There are many nuggets of practical information for parents and caregivers nestled within the various studies reviewed here.

Several enhancements could profitably extend investigations on the socialization of emotion. Use of even more naturalistic, home-based techniques, such as observing real emotional interchanges and conversations about real emotions between children and their mothers *and fathers*, would be useful (Dunn, Brown, Slomkowski, et al., 1991; Fivush, 1989). Such direct observation would allow researchers to delineate more conclusively the relations among parental encouragement/discouragement of children's expressiveness; children's expression of and attention to parental emotions; and their subsequent expression, understanding, and reaction to emotions. Moreover, future research should include indicators of parents' degree and intensity of expressiveness, so that the contribution of these more qualitative views of emotionality can be assessed. And the contributions of other socializers with whom preschoolers spend much time, including preschool and day care teachers, older siblings, and even peers, remain almost unknown.

More attention also needs to be paid to the direction of effects in the emotion socialization system. Parents differentially socialize children, depending on their emotional competence (Denham et al., 1992; Eisenberg & Fabes, 1994). They probably tailor socialization techniques for children who are more or less emotionally competent. An interactional or transactional perspective would be more productive in specifying the development of emotional expressiveness and understanding. Intentionally focusing on both children's and parents' contributions to these aspects of emotional competence could result in a more complicated, but truer, picture of the development of emotional compete.

Expansion of these lines of research across longitudinal periods would allow investigators to tease out the direction of effects through the use of structural modeling techniques. Such expanded longitudinal research could also make possible more extensive examination of interactions between child sex or age and parental socialization techniques, as well as the possibility of nonlinear relations between children's and parents' expressed emotions and emotion understanding.[5]

## NOTES

1. Although the mother–child relationship made bidirectionality of effects almost certain here (mothers with whiny, fussy children become more frustrated and negative themselves!) the maternal emotion displays during lunch and the "doctor's" visit were correlated with children's emotions in situations where the mothers were absent, even after children's emotions during lunch and the "doctor's" visit were accounted for. This finding suggests that, over and above a possible bidirectional effect of children's own emotions, maternal emotions contribute to children's ability to marshal emotional resources in independent situations.

2. As I have noted in Chapter 2, there is some controversy about whether young children actually experience certain emotions, notably shame and guilt.

3. Hyson and Lee (1996) are working to devise a measure of early childhood teachers' attitudes about their impact on emotional competence, including a scale on direct teaching about emotion. We have promising preliminary results on the importance of fathers' emotion language (Denham, Mitchell-Copeland, et al., 1997), and Dunn et al. (1987) shed some light on the contributions of sibling emotion conversation.

4. Fathers' inconsistency, on the other hand, was marginally negatively related to children's understanding of emotional situations. This finding highlights the need to obtain information from both parents.

5. For example, an inverted-U function might be proposed for the relation between some aspects of parental negative emotion and emotion understanding: Mothers who show no anger all *or* very much anger may have children who are similarly lacking in comprehension.

# Chapter 5

# Emotion Regulation

$P$reschoolers are learning to regulate their own emotions. Various strategies to regulate emotions surface during the preschool period. One is self-talk.

*Emily repeats emotion language her parents have used with her, to help herself calm down: "Big kids like Emmy and Carl and Linda don't cry. THEY big kids . . . the baby cry at Tanta's . . . babies can cry but . . . big kids like Emmy don't cry . . . they go sleep . . . " (Engel, 1995, p. 39).*

*Similarly, Ella has twisted her ankle while dancing on the patio. The discomfort wakes her in the night, and her mother comforts her and talks to her about what is bothering her. She asks whether she should kiss the hurt foot. "No, I'll do it," Ella replies. She lies back down in bed, holds her foot, and whispers over and over to herself, "Nice and better. Nice and better." Soon she is asleep.*

Both girls successfully regulate their emotions.

An important part of emotional competence is emotion regulation (hereafter abbreviated as ER). Emotions can be stressful: Negative, but also positive, emotions can exceed children's resources. They slowly seep into, or even flood, their conscious awareness. When this happens, the children's behavior and/or thought processes can become disor-

147

ganized, instigating a need for ER (Barrett & Campos, 1991; Eisenberg & Fabes, 1992). But not all toddlers and preschoolers are as capable of managing emotions as Emily and Ella:

> *Two-year-old Chuckie, tired and hungry already, demands that his mother turn on the television as she tries to stow groceries in the kitchen cupboard. Upon receiving a curt "Not now," he begins to cry, thrashing and kicking on the kitchen floor. What can he do? He wants his show right now, but Mom looks mad, too.*

> *Three-year-old Melissa is approached by a Rottweiler and cringes in fear. What are her options?*

> *Four-year-old Roberta is playing "chase" on the playground with a large group of buddies. Together, they laugh hard and loud, over and over, until they fall to the ground in a heap. As their preschool teacher calls to them, they are still chuckling and slapping at each other; they don't even hear her.*

ER plays a role in each of these situations. In this chapter, I first try to create a successful working definition for ER; I then describe strategies that constitute its affective, cognitive, and behavioral components. I also elucidate factors that moderate children's developing abilities to regulate emotions, and discuss the socialization of these important aspects of emotional competence.

Emotional arousal is unavoidable. Children and adults alike register emotion at all times. Negative emotions need to be managed especially often. There are many ways to modulate emotion—to minimize its expression and experience, as called for in the three examples above. People learn ways to tolerate and endure experiences of emotions that are just a bit "too much"; this modulation, toleration, and endurance of emotions are the essence of ER (see Kopp, 1989).

Sometimes, too, the experience and/or expression of emotion need to be "up-regulated"—"whistling a happy tune" when afraid, showing more anger than is felt in order to "win," or crying piteously to obtain help. Usually when ER is discussed, however, much more emphasis is put on the "down-regulating" of emotions. This distinction is probably a fair one, because I think that down-regulation is more often necessary than up-regulation. In this chapter, I most often follow this line of thinking. Nonetheless, it is important to consider situations where augmentation of emotional experience and expression is important.

Clearly, preschoolers are already working at all of this. Even very young children begin to deal with the stress caused by emotions and emotional situations, and to consider managing emotions through both down- and up-regulation. In fact, despite their legendary negative reactions to others' discomfort and to conflict-laden environments (see, e.g., Cummings et al., 1981), even infants and toddlers are already beginning to try to deal with their emotions. For example, 3-month-old infants exposed to mothers' flat or depressed affect demonstrate negative affect of their own, but they also show various behaviors that may be precursors of more sophisticated attempts at coping, such as sucking on a pacifier or averting their gaze (Tronick, 1989). Eighteen-month-olds self-soothe when their mothers are absent (Garner, 1995). Regardless of age, ER occurs constantly in some form or other: Whether consciously or unconsciously, people are aware of and are fine-tuning their emotional experience and expression (Bridges & Grolnick, 1995; see also the "self-monitoring" path in Chapter 1, Figure 1.1).

## DEFINING EMOTION REGULATION

The concept of ER is a slippery one to define and operationalize, however. Many highly regarded investigators in developmental psychology continue to struggle with this task. It is hard to capture the essence of ER because it is really inextricable from experiencing and expressing emotions, and is to some degree allied with the understanding of emotions. Accordingly, I return to a functionalist definition of emotions themselves in the effort to delineate ER more clearly: "Emotions, from a functionalist perspective, equal the attempts by the person to establish, maintain, change, or terminate the relationship between the person and environment in matters of significance" (Campos, Mumme, Kermoian, & Campos, 1994, p. 28).

In the three examples above, Chuckie is trying to change a personally important aspect of the environment—he wants his cartoons! Melissa wants to get rid of the dog. And Roberta is having difficulty maintaining the state of fun with friends without being overwhelmed by it. In each example, the experience and expression of emotion become too strong or too long-lasting for the child and/or his or her social partners. ER, then, is needed when internal resources are exceeded, or when the child's own expectations or those of others are not met. In more abstract terms, and to admit the possibility of up-regulation, ER is necessary when either the presence or absence of emotional expression and experience interferes with a person's goals.

Another issue needing attention when one is trying to define ER is that, as Thompson (1993) has asserted, ER has been regarded both as an outcome and as a process. He suggests the following definition: "Emotion regulation consists of the extrinsic and intrinsic processes responsible for *monitoring, evaluating, and modifying* emotional reactions, especially their intensive and temporal features, to accomplish one's goals" (Thompson, 1994, pp. 27–28; emphasis added). When we use this perspective as a lens with which to view ER, it becomes clear that some of the definitional difficulty is that investigators are looking at differing angles of the phenomenon, much like the blind men describing the elephant in the old fable. Just as the functional viewpoint suggests that there are specific patterns of expressiveness for all emotions, particular behavioral action tendencies, and cognitive goals associated with them (Barrett & Campos, 1991), there are also emotional, cognitive, and behavioral aspects of ER—the "monitoring, evaluating, and modifying" to which Thompson refers. To tell the full story about its development, all of these aspects must be pursued.

## THE COMPONENTS OF EMOTION REGULATION

The key components of ER incorporate these three dimensions—emotional, cognitive, and behavioral. Figure 5.1 depicts my view of the multifaceted nature of ER. The emotional dimension of ER is marked by self-soothing physiological arousal. The cognitive dimension of ER includes refocusing attention and problem-solving reasoning. The "behavioral" aspects of ER encompass modifying expressions, thoughts, or behaviors related to the emotional experience (and can thus be emotional, cognitive, or behavioral; see below), as well as getting organized for coordinated action in the service of one's goal (Gottman & Katz, 1989; Miller & Green, 1985).

My view of ER is directly related to the definition of emotion I have put forward in Chapter 1. Each of the steps of emotional experience—emotional arousal, cognitive construal, and behavioral action—can require regulation, and thus is a part of ER. As stated there, and as shown in Figure 1.1, both emotional experience and ER involve the following steps:

1. Emotional arousal is experienced and monitored: What are the sensations like?
2. Often almost simultaneously, the child perceptually and cognitively considers the situation: What do these sensations mean to me?
3. Finally, he or she chooses specific responses that serve the goal of modulating emotional experience: What can I do, if anything, about

these emotional experiences I have discerned? Do I need to act, and if so, how?

Thus, although emotional arousal can incapacitate a child's abilities to think and act, the experience of emotion can also help a child organize adaptive processes through cognitive processes and behavioral attempts at coping. Figure 5.1 shows my conception of these components.

## Emotional Component

The first component of ER, then, is distinctly emotional. I would agree with Thompson (1994) that people must keep track of, as well as modify, the actual experience of emotion. Even young children are probably beginning to monitor the temporal and intensive features of emotion. They are aware of their arousal (see the leftmost columns of Figures 1.1 and Figure 5.1), though not necessarily consciously. As they are beginning to appreciate sensory information and to articulate the nature of their own sensory functioning (O'Neill, Astington, & Flavell, 1992; Weinberger & Bushnell, 1994), they probably start to appreciate aspects of their own emotions, albeit imperfectly. They sense how

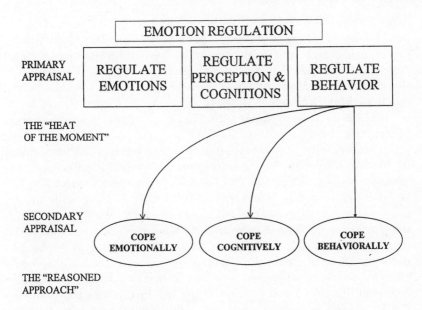

**FIGURE 5.1.** Model of emotion regulation (ER).

strongly they feel an emotion, how quickly it comes upon them, and when and how it peaks.

In the three examples above, temporal and intensive features of the emotions experienced overburden each child's immediate ability to organize thinking and behavior. Two-year-old Chuckie's quick latency and rise time for anger, along with its intensity, make his wanting his way (and his mother's afternoon!) quite difficult. Three-year-old Melissa's persistent fear leaves her shaky even after the dog moves on. And 4-year-old Roberta, though happy and ostensibly enjoying a positive experience with her friends, takes a long time to recover from the high-intensity experience; she acts and feels out of control.

Unfortunately, few researchers have focused on the temporal and intensive features of emotions; this state of affairs continues, in my view, because psychology only recently became able to operationalize emotions comfortably at all. Nonetheless, highlighting these aspects of emotional experience should prove important. Adults, peers, and the children themselves must ascertain as much as possible about the particular emotion that a child is experiencing in order to predict whether ER is necessary, and, if so, its likely means.

## Cognitive/Perceptual Component

After acknowledging the feelings being experienced, the second important aspect of ER is a cognitive/perceptual one. The child who is experiencing and monitoring emotion has at his or her disposal perceptual and cognitive ways of managing the situation. These include the child's external or internal means of redeploying attention when emotion either becomes "too much" or seems "too little," as well as his or her initial interpretations of the emotionally arousing events (Thompson, 1994).

The decision to pay attention or not to an emotional situation and its attendant arousal—that is, setting up an "emotions gatekeeper"—is primarily perceptual. Both a child and a caregiver can control whether an emotional situation is perceived at all. A child can internally change the attention given to emotion-eliciting stimuli: When confronted with the Rottweiler, Melissa may go into an almost dissociative state if the fear is severe enough—sucking her finger, closing her eyes, looking as if she is asleep. In contrast, external means of refocusing a child's attention are often attempted by adults: Roberta's teacher may separate her from the crowd and attempt to get her involved in more low-key activity. At this perceptual level, the child calibrates how much of the emotional experience leaks into awareness—from totally ignoring the emotion to being focused upon it to the exclusion of all else.

When attention must be directed toward the emotional situation, it cannot be totally ignored or neutralized. At this cognitive level, children not only "take in" emotions, but figure them out at a very elemental level. Instead of internally or externally avoiding the elicitor of the emotion, or becoming fixated upon it, children can interpret the situation. Intensity, duration, rise time, and latency of emotion all signal the success or failure of their goals. Their subsequent cognitive appreciations of how these aspects of their emotional experience relate to their goals aid preschoolers in seeking to diminish or augment a particular emotional experience.

In keeping with the model of emotion presented in Figure 1.1, children make fundamental decisions, which I would call "primary appraisals," of the personal significance of the person–environment encounters signaled by emotion: "I have something at stake; something bad [or good] is happening that matters to me." (See the middle of Figure 1.1, and also Figure 5.1.) They then evaluate the situation's features and its potential for fitting with their goals (Eisenberg & Fabes, 1992; Folkman, 1991). In the examples above, Chuckie sees that he is not going to get something he desires; Melissa is aware that she is going to get something she does *not* desire; and Roberta sees that she is getting something she desires, but that it is going slightly awry.

But these interpretations could have been different, with very dissimilar implications for the regulations of these children's emotional experience and expressiveness. As he watches his mother, Chuckie could decide that stacking the boxes and cans of food on a low shelf is fun and feel more interest than anger. He may even get a cookie out of this! Melissa may notice the 6-year-old walking along with the Rottweiler and interpret her arousal as joy at being united with an old friend and her *new* dog. Roberta may consider her extreme hilarity a signal of interference with her goal of bodily safety (almost feeling pain from all the laughing) and retreat to a quiet corner of the playground. Similarly, the little girl about to recite a poem (see Chapter 2) could see her "butterflies" as excitement rather than fear. What is important here is that arousal needs a name, and the immediate "spin" put on physiological signs of emotions may render them more or less palatable.

These first two steps of ER—emotional monitoring and perceptual/cognitive evaluating—are often quite inextricable. The means of perceptually controlling attention and cognitively "figuring out" the situation are central to children's experience of emotion itself, and often occur nearly simultaneously (for more information on this aspect of ER, see Barrett & Campos, 1991; Campos, Campos, & Barrett, 1989; Stein & Trabasso, 1989; Thompson, 1994; Thompson & Calkins, 1996).

These steps can take place very quickly. What happens next, if an individual has any time for reflection, is much more influenced by the cortical areas of the brain, and can proceed more thoughtfully. Consequently, most behavioral ER is more reflective and is related to coping[1]: What can *I* do about this arousal I have interpreted?

## "Behavioral" Component: Coping

Strategies to deal directly with the experienced and interpreted emotion, its causes and consequences, constitute the next component of ER. The child's next step, after first experiencing the emotion and quickly making a primary appraisal of the situation, is making another fundamental decision about the options for coping (or what I would call a "secondary appraisal" of): "Given this feeling, [what emotion is it, and] what can I *do* about it?" (See the rightmost columns of Figures 1.1 and 5.1.)

But *doing* something need not be overt and active. Coping responses themselves—the "doing something" aspect of ER—can be emotional, cognitive, or behavioral. Coping changes one's arousal level and other temporal features of the emotion experienced in that situation (as in the self-monitoring path in Figure 1.1), the focus of one's attention in the situation, one's goal for the situation, the expressive pattern shown, or the problem situation itself. That is, "behavioral" responses of ER can include facial, vocal, or physiological expressive responses, cognitive reappraisals, or enactment of behavioral strategies. I think that this multifaceted nature of coping perplexes researchers who are trying to get a grip on ER. Hence, there are emotional, cognitive/perceptual, and behavioral aspects of ER, but there are also emotional, cognitive/perceptual, and behavioral means of coping within the "behavioral" component of ER. This overlap is, I feel, the source of much confusion.[2] Coping, the endpoint of "optimal" ER, varies according to these dimensions, which are tied tightly to the particular child's goals in the particular situation.

### Emotional Coping

The function of emotional coping is to change expressive behavior, in order to change both the expression and experience of emotion. Controlling emotional responses helps the child avoid overarousal: The child can try to modulate the intensity, rise time, threshold, or latency of the emotion as expressed, or even to alter the discrete emotion being expressed. These efforts at coping feed back to the original state of arousal, subtly or not so subtly changing it.

Minimizing emotional expression is not the only viable means of emotional coping in the service of ER. The capacity for generating and sustaining emotions can also be important, because accentuated emotional responses can function as social regulators, especially to gain help or get one's way. A sad preschooler cries out loud when his or her mother appears, because this choice of behavior is directly related to receiving comfort.

The choice of expressive coping responses which allow the child to continue showing emotion in accordance with his or her goals also depends strongly on the context of the emotion experience, and thus is often situation-specific (Thompson, 1994). The child's individual expressive repertoire, his or her goals, the demands of the setting, and the values of social partners all interact. If she is accompanied by someone who will laugh at her, Melissa wants to diminish the intensity of her expression of fear of the Rottweiler, or at least to increase its latency. She seeks to diminish her expression and experience of fear if she is alone, but to enhance her expression of fear if an adult is nearby and can rush to her aid. If Mom looks really annoyed at his outburst, Chuckie does not stop feeling angry altogether, but he tries to rein in the intensity of his expressed anger. Instead of screaming, he forcefully glares at his mother in order to change her mind by dint of his mighty will!

## Cognitive Coping

Cognitive coping steps are also possible: Children can relinquish the goal they have identified in the perceptual/cognitive ER step. They may also purposefully choose a new goal, or think through new causal attributions that help them feel more comfortable in their world. A preschool boy who is sad about not going swimming may say to himself, "I didn't want to go anyway." Roberta may decide she is tired of running around and would prefer to swing alone for a while. Melissa may decide that the Rottweiler is approaching because he wants to be her friend. In addition, the cognitive activity of pretend play can allow a preschooler to defuse anxiety through practice at solving problems, comforting self-talk, or other means (L. A. Barnett, 1984).

For this type of coping, too, there are context effects. Importantly, the particular emotion elicited by the situation helps govern likely modes of coping. Self-conscious and social emotions (e.g., guilt and shame) may require mostly cognitive coping, such as rationalizing, "I'll be a good boy so I won't feel bad any more." These difficult and complex emotions can also be dealt with by downplaying the importance of other people's opinions, the wrongdoing, or the enviable person or possession. Similarly, discerning that high-level happiness calls for ER can require a preschooler to be cognitively and perceptually aware of subtle contextual nuances—for instance, that a level of glee appropriate to the playground is not okay in the preschool classroom.

### Behavioral Coping

Children also *do* things to cope with the experience of emotion. Again, the emotion being experienced helps to determine the behavioral coping effort chosen. As an example, people do different things to cope with anger as opposed to fear. With anger, the possibilities are to strike, argue, or retreat; with fear, the prominent coping alternatives are to self-soothe or seek comfort from others. Furthermore, regulation of such emotions as sadness, anger, and fear requires the most active behavioral strategies, which help the child to suppress, modulate, or even augment the emotions' action tendencies. A 5-year-old boy crying over losing a game tries to stop his whimpering because he doesn't want to feel bad or be ridiculed. Minutes later he may purposely roar very loudly at the "ex"-friend he supposedly caught cheating; he accentuates his anger to get his way.

### "Optimal" Coping

Clearly, after a child experiences an emotion (performing the emotional step of ER), then attends to it and figures it out (performing the cognitive step of ER), there are a lot of "behavioral," or coping, choices. Some choices are undoubtedly more satisfying than others. What satisfies the child experiencing the emotion, however, may not please the other people in his or her social group at the time. As always, the personal experience of emotion *and* the social expression of emotion must be considered. For instance, the 5-year-old who lost the game may feel smug when he deals with his anger by hitting the "cheater"; undoubtedly, though, the "cheater" does not consider this choice so successful! Melissa may retreat from the dog and suck her thumb on the edge of the playground; although this helps her to regain her equilibrium, her mother worries that she is *too* scared of things, too uninvolved.

In addition to depending on who is involved, the success of coping is related to temporal factors. Short-term success is not necessarily accompanied by long-term success. A preschooler may have no "best" routes to regulating the expression and experience of emotions. For example, the daughter of a depressed mother may choose to soothe both her own and her mother's sadness and fear by comforting the mother and enacting behaviors that are very empathic on the surface. But there can be a long-term price to pay for this mode of ER (Thompson & Calkins, 1996; see also Chapter 7). So there is often no "optimal" means of coping, whether emotional, cognitive, or behavioral (Thompson & Calkins, 1996).

## DEVELOPMENTAL TRAJECTORY AND INDIVIDUAL DIFFERENCES IN EMOTION REGULATION

As for all developmental phenomena, the important questions to ask about ER are "What changes?" and "What stays the same?" Accordingly, in the sections that follow I review changes in supported and independent ER during the preschool age range.[3] At first, adults need to support young children's ER efforts; little by little, though, preschoolers usually gain some independent means to regulate emotions.

Age change and stability are not the whole picture, however. Individual differences are important as well. Children differ in the types of ER they manifest in the "same" situation, and particular ER processes may or may not succeed in increasing the adaptiveness of a particular child's functioning (Barrett & Campos, 1991). Individual differences in ER and their socialization must also be explored. Thus, I not only explore the changes in ER from toddlerhood through the preschool age, but describe the nature and source of some individual differences.

### Developmental Change in Strategies for ER

Because of its complexity as an emotional, cognitive, and behavioral entity, ER consists of loosely connected abilities with differing timetables (Thompson, 1994). In general, adult support in ER is often needed in the toddler and early preschool years. Then children become increasingly adept at using their own independent ER strategies.

#### Supported ER Strategies

Caregivers are very important to the inception of ER. Toddlers and young preschoolers often need external support to become skilled at regulating their emotions (Kopp, 1989; Maccoby, 1983; Thompson, 1994); their parents' and caregivers' support allows their ER strategies to be maximally effective.

Early in the toddler-to-preschool period, parents often assist their children in a cognitive coping strategy they will come to use themselves—that is, purposely redeploying attention. This can be a very useful means of regulating emotion. Specific ER strategies are demonstrated by parents and caregivers as well, and may be learned by children. In one study, children whose mothers used comforting, instrumental, cognitive, and distraction ER strategies were more likely to use the same strategy types as their mothers (Stansbury & Sigman, 1995). Caregivers and parents can also structure a child's environment for a better fit with the child's ER abilities. One mother chooses not to walk down a certain path while enjoying a spring stroll because she sees a large dog that will frighten her daughter. Another father avoids arranging a play date with a certain child who he knows will leave his son cranky and overstimulated.

Emotion language is an especially powerful tool for ER because it allows children to state their feelings, to understand feedback on them, and to process causal associations between events and emotions, thus enabling the choice of a coping response (Kopp, 1989). Preschoolers with access to more sophisticated maternal emotion language during emotion discussion and simulation coped more productively with their own emotions expressed in their preschool classroom (Denham et al., 1992; see similar results for children of depressed mothers in Zahn-Waxler, Ridgeway, Denham, Usher, & Cole, 1993, as discussed in Chapter 7). Talk about emotions with parents can enable preschoolers to stay on a more emotionally positive even keel in other situations (see also Chapter 4). Conversations about emotion play a prominent role in parents' frequent reconstruing or recasting of emotionally arousing events: How many preschoolers have heard the words "This will only hurt a little"?

### Children as Partners in ER

Thus, during toddlerhood parents take the lead in assisting ER, but even during this early period an individual child is likely to make some independent efforts toward ER. As the preschool period progresses, adult support is still important, but ER is more and more a partnership as children become simultaneously more autonomous and more capable of cooperation.

Even toddlers can use a few independent ER schemes, such as orientation of attention toward or away from a stimulus, self-distraction via physical self-comforting or self-stimulation, approaching or retreating from a situation, or cognitive and symbolic manipulations of a situation through play (Kopp, 1989). Shatz (1994) reports on the ability of her 2-year-old grandson, Ricky, to distance or disengage in order to gain control over his emotions:

I offered [Ricky] a banana and opened the peel just a little. Ricky's habit was to pull the peel down a bit at a time as he ate the banana, but this night he pulled the peel down too far at once. Annoyed, he tried to throw the banana on the floor, but I intervened . . . there was no compromising. Ricky was angry. He climbed down from his chair and went to stand in a corner facing the wall. . . . After about ten minutes Richard . . . found him lying on the couch in the TV room. R: [Grouchily]: Don't bodder me. I sleeping. (p. 129)

After toddlerhood, young children slowly build up associations between ER efforts—usually coping efforts, be they emotional, cognitive, or behavioral—and concomitant changes in their feeling states. Their exclusive reliance on caregivers' help with ER lessens, and their ·awareness of the need for coping strategies increases (Maccoby, 1983). They come to appreciate the success or failure of their attempts at ER, and become more flexible in choosing the most optimal ways of coping in specific contexts. Behavioral disorganization resulting from strong negative affect decreases, probably because of this concomitantly increasing repertoire of emotional, cognitive, and behavioral coping strategies relevant to an expanding sphere of situations (Cole, Michel, & Teti, 1994). These independent ER strategies available to preschoolers increase primarily as a function of cognitive development and socialization. The influence of cognitive development can be seen in the following ways:

- The number and variety of emotions that can be understood (see also Chapter 3).
- The number and variety of the child's coping responses.
- The child's ability to modulate his or her emotions consciously (see also Chapter 2), via the following:

    Feeling rules ("Big kids don't get upset when their parents leave").

    Display rules ("Don't show that emotion, or show it *this* way").

    Coping rules ("When you are afraid, whistle a happy tune to distract yourself").

What are these independent coping strategies of behavioral ER? First, some coping strategies focus on changing the emotion being experienced (Folkman, 1991)—for example, whispering "Nice and better." Other emotional coping strategies used during the preschool period include venting, avoidance, and expressing dislike/disapproval (Fabes & Eisenberg, 1992).

Some coping strategies are predominantly perceptual or cognitive.

Preschoolers become able to regulate emotional experience via paying attention to nondistressing aspects of the environment, rather than fixating on more distressing elements (Bridges & Grolnick, 1994, 1995; Grolnick, Bridges, & Connell, 1996; Grolnick, McMenamy, Kurowski, & Bridges, 1997). These children's cognitive coping via distraction then moves into more behavioral coping: Their active engagement with the environment involves play with toys, general exploration, or engaging another person (via smiles, showing toys, vocalizing, or inviting the other to play).

Preschoolers can also find a new goal, or revise what they consider the causes of their own emotions—for instance, "I want to use these Legos instead of these wooden blocks," or "No, Mom, I'm sad because my tummy hurts [not because my friend took my toy]." Another cognitive way for a child to influence the conditions necessitating ER is simply to maximize his or her fit with conditions as they are; active change is sometimes impossible. After the preschool period, coping strategies become increasingly cognitive and less dependent on observable behaviors, in situations such as a friend's moving away, another kid's saying a mean thing, waiting for an injection, or experiencing an adult's anger (Band & Weisz, 1988). Older children can "think about" rather than "do" something else.

The third way to influence the conditions necessitating ER is problem-focused, usually a behavioral means of actively changing the emotion-inducing situation (e.g., turning the page when there is a scary picture in a book). Behavioral coping strategies used by preschoolers in response to their own anger include revenge, active resistance, and adult seeking (Fabes & Eisenberg, 1992). Although both cognitive and behavioral ER strategies are used throughout the preschool period, behavioral means still outpace cognitive (Band & Weisz, 1988). Instrumental strategies—doing something to fix the eliciting situation or alleviate obstacles—predominate (Strayer & Schroeder, 1989).

At quite an early age, children become sensitive to context-dependent features of adaptive ER processes. They know when the support of their parents is available or unavailable; the young preschoolers in Grolnick et al.'s (1996) research most often used active engagement of another person to aid them in ER when their mothers were present and not preoccupied. They did not seek comfort when the experimenter had asked their mothers to be preoccupied with a magazine.

No matter which means of ER a child uses in a particular situation, it is important for them to feel that they have control over their own ER. No one likes feeling "out of control." Children aged 5 and 6 who watched a scary fairy tale on videotape, and did not believe they had control over frightening events, remembered less of a subsequent videotape on children's medical examinations (Cortez & Bugental, 1994). They felt the need to assert some measure of control, and subsequently used attentional disengagement during the second video to lessen their short-term distress. Using this mode of ER exacted a price, however: Through its use, they were insufficiently attentive and acquired only limited useful knowledge of a potentially threatening but ubiquitous event—a medical examination.

Children who feel that they have little control over ER also vent their emotions (with varying results, depending on the target of the venting), or even sublimate through illness, compensating activity, or dissociation (Cole, Michel, & Teti, 1994; Miller & Green, 1985). Obviously, the lack of ER has varying deleterious effects, including inability to acquire important information, alienation of potential sources of support, and relative loss of contact with reality. These findings highlight the need to teach ER to children who need such support.

### Moderators of Independent ER Strategy Usage

Even within the preschool range, age and gender moderate types of ER strategies chosen, especially for coping with anger. After experiencing anger in the preschool classroom, younger boys are more likely to show overt anger and seek escape than other age/sex groups are; older girls are more likely to actively resist the thing or person that causes their anger, as well as less likely to seek adults to cope (Fabes & Eisenberg, 1992).

Similarly, when 3- and 4-year-olds were asked to refrain from playing with a group of special toys, and not allowed to eat a snack already available, the younger group used more instrumental strategies to help them ease their frustration—stating or restating their reasonable requests, or just getting or doing the desired thing (Stansbury & Sigman, 1995). The 4-year-olds used more cognitive strategies than the 3-year-olds did.

### Awareness of ER Strategies

When during the preschool period do children become aware of their increasingly sophisticated strategies for coping with their own and others' emotions? Ability to reflect on ER strategies would seem likely to predict more optimal ER. In Chapter 3, the development of children's understanding of how to change emotions has been described. In general, preschoolers seem to know much about direct and indirect means to change sadness and anger. They have some limited understanding of how to make a happy person feel "just okay," but young children's knowledge about *augmentation* of happiness has not been assessed, to my knowledge.

It is important to note, however, that most of this work has focused on what young children think can be done to change another person's emotions. If, as I argue, the behavioral "piece" of ER is in the selection of coping strategies, knowing what children think about their *own* ER is vital. But few studies focus on it. Part of the obstacle here is, of course, the difficulty of asking children about internal experience.

Direct questioning about ER can yield some intriguing findings. When asked, "What's the thing to do when you're feeling depressed?", children aged 4 to 11 mostly mentioned play strategies or actually doing something fun to feel better; fewer children endorsed avoidance strategies or seeking help and comfort (Kenealy, 1989). In a similar vein, children were asked what they would do when negative events befell them, or what others should do in negative situations. Kindergartners, more often than second-graders, reported social support and seeking adult help as ER solutions; this focus was appropriate because kindergartners need, and more often experience, supported ER (Bernzweig, Eisenberg, & Fabes, 1993; see also Altshuler & Ruble, 1989; Beaver, 1997). Older children suggested more direct problem-solving and cognitive strategies. The age change in these self-reported strategies parallels observational findings.

Apparently young children do have some awareness of their own ER methods. Clearly, though, this area is ready for exploration. If more engaging methodologies were presented to preschoolers, even more illuminating results might emerge regarding changes in internal and external manifestations of emotion, construals of emotions, and coping behaviors. Story methods, for example, could be used, as they are in research on understanding of emotions. Recently Halpern (1997) has reported on a method that at least gets at coping behavior. Preschoolers were told stories about dealing with their feelings during a peer conflict, a mother–child conflict, a mastery problem, and a scary time. Then they were asked what to do in these emotionally charged scenarios; their responses fell into the categories of problem-focused solutions, venting, avoidance, acceptance, and lack of strategy. The new method's validity is demonstrated by significant relations between strategy deficiency and internalizing symptoms. Perhaps even more ingeniously, a mixture of observational and interview methods could be utilized to ask children who show specific emotions how they would regulate them—either in real time or, perhaps more advantageously, at a later videotape review.

## Individual Differences in ER during the Preschool Period

As Halpern (1997) has recently uncovered, even preschoolers differ in their patterns of ER. When exposed to the anger of others, for example, young children may freeze, make a distress face, show gestural/postural distress, try to shut out or escape the background anger, watch intently, express verbal concern to the antagonists, cry, or even smile (Cummings, 1987). How can such variation in individual responding be explained? Over and above developmental differences in ER, it is vital to explain these individual differences.

Eisenberg and Fabes (1992) have developed a model of ER in early childhood that promises to aid the search for differing patterns of ER from child to child. These authors posit that two important temperamental dimensions must be assessed to predict the ER strategies used by young children. These temperamental elements underlie, and may either facilitate or disrupt, coping attempts:

- Stable individual differences in parameters of emotional intensity, such as threshold and rise time.
- Stable individual differences in regulatory processes, such as attentional shifting or focusing, and voluntary initiation or inhibition of action.

An individual child's relative standing on these two characteristics determines how successful his or her ER is in social situations, and how it is received by important persons in the social environment. Furthermore, the centrality of these characteristics makes sense because they map onto the emotional, cognitive, and behavioral steps of ER.

One possible combination of these two characteristics will result in a very intense but also highly regulated individual. Highly intense but also very regulated children appear shy, withdrawn, inhibited, and unable to enjoy social situations. A child who is low in emotional intensity but nonetheless very regulated may appear affectively "flat" and unsociable, for example (Eisenberg, Bernzweig, & Fabes, 1991).

Intensity coupled with low regulation is even more problematic. Unbridled intensity of emotional reactivity is clearly often associated with difficulties in ER. Preschoolers with less positive moods outside conflict situations are more likely to cope with conflict through aggressive venting or acting out (Arsenio & Lover, 1997; Eisenberg et al., 1993). Emotional intensity and negative affect are also related to acting-out means of coping with emotion; for boys, such expressiveness is also negatively associated with constructive coping, such as verbal objections and leaving the situation (Eisenberg et al., 1993,

1994). Moreover, children of high emotional intensity, especially high-intensity anger, react to adult anger with increased distress, negative appraisals, and aggression (Cummings et al., 1985; Davies & Cummings, 1995). Finally, mothers' reports of low emotional intensity are related to children's use of nonabusive language to deal with anger, whereas their ratings of their children's negative emotionality (sadness and fear) are associated with escape behaviors observed during children's anger in preschool (Eisenberg et al., 1994). Overall, these associations make intuitive sense; "hotheads" are not commonly expected to be able to deal with emotion-provoking situations in a constructive manner.

The moderately regulated, moderately emotionally intense child is probably in the best position to succeed at ER. Such a child is emotionally expressive, but also capable of planning, problem-focused coping, and flexible use of various ER strategies. All told, this model for individual differences in ER looks very promising. More specific operationalization and testing of the control component need to be pursued.

Furthermore, it may be that not only the level of arousal (i.e., emotional intensity) is important to ER. Valence of prevalent emotion may also be relevant: Davies and Cummings (1995) found that children induced to experience positive emotions were less distressed and held more positive cognitions while experiencing background anger. Inclusion of a third factor, level of emotion understanding, could make the model even more complete.

This model of individual differences in ER, with its emphasis on temperament, points to the likelihood of biological contributions to ER and emotional competence as a whole. Nonetheless, I subscribe to a more inclusive view of the etiology of emotional competence, in which both biological (species-typical, genetic, and physiological) factors and social factors interweave in a complex medley. Thus, I now turn to socialization of individual differences in ER.

## Socialization of Individual Differences in Preschoolers' ER

So, although the pivotal aspects of Eisenberg and Fabes's (1992) model are related to temperament, the contribution of socialization to ER is still important. Consonant with the general state of ER conceptualization and research, much remains to be learned about its socialization. The model of parental socialization of emotion, including modeling, contingency, and coaching (this component of the model has been mentioned earlier), is a good place to start in considering parental contributors to young children's ER.

*Parents' Own Emotions and ER*

The profiles of emotions displayed by parents can be very important to the socialization of children's coping with their own and others' emotions. And, as mentioned in my discussion of supported ER, socializers model ways of dealing with emotions. Some parents teach their children to hide or suppress their emotions, but others emphasize such coping techniques as direct problem solving or seeking social support (Eisenberg et al., 1992; Roberts & Strayer, 1987).

So far, though, few studies have looked at the relation between parents' own emotions or ER and children's ER efforts. Garner (1995) did find that mothers who reported more positive emotion in their families had toddlers who were more capable of self-soothing when they were absent. And, if one possible endpoint of ER is an emotional profile with greater positive than negative emotionality, my work supports the hypothesis that parents model ER (Denham, 1989; Denham & Grout, 1992, 1993): The children of parents who are well regulated have a well-balanced emotional profile likewise. Of course, these studies also hint at the possibility of intergenerational similarities in biologically based temperaments.

*Parents' Coaching about Emotions*

I see ER at the intersection of expressiveness, understanding, and socialization. "Emotions happen for these reasons [understanding]. This is how they are experienced and expressed [expressiveness]. We parents expect you to use your understanding to help deal with your emotional experiences." Coaching about emotions adds to children's understanding generally, in terms of where and why emotions occur (see Chapter 4), but also more particularly in terms of how they are to be expressed. So, given this view of ER, coaching should be a particularly valuable aspect of its socialization. Unfortunately, however, I know of no empirical research that directly addresses the impact of coaching on ER.

Nonetheless, Thompson (1990) posits several ways in which parents' verbal discourse or conversations with children contribute to ER. First, there are direct commands and instructions about emotions—the guiding and socializing language that my colleagues and I measure in examining children and parents' naturally occurring discourse and reminiscing about emotions. Parents constantly try to aid their children in approximating cultural and family norms about the expression of emotions: "Stop that crying!" "We don't laugh at people like that when we beat them at games. It's so mean!" Though it varies across families, this socialization pressure is always present to one degree or another, and is made explicit verbally.

Sometimes parents not only state the rules of expressiveness, but also suggest clear means of performing ER. As good coaches, they try to weigh the potential effect of stressful circumstances, and then to think of solutions.

*Will the waiting-room time at a father's own doctor's office be just a bit too long for Carlos to tolerate? The father thinks it may be. He suggests that Carlos look at a book as a distraction.*

*With her two children in tow, a mother remembers their last visit to her own mother as she pulls into the parking space in front of the house. Wisely, she not only tells Sophie and Sebastian, "You need to be kind to Grandma and not fuss about how you can't get good channels on her television," but also helps them redefine goals: "You might feel less frustrated if you don't even try to watch TV at Grandma's house. I'll bet it would be more fun to use her swing in the back yard."*

Parents suggest the full complement of ER strategies at one time or another.

Less direct discussions, about parents' own emotions, affect children's ER by shaping the children's conceptions of emotion in general and of "big people's" ER strategies in particular. Is it normal to feel anger in a wide range of social interactions? In one of these situations, would it be perfectly okay to punch a hole in the wall? As seen in preceding chapters, preschoolers are keen observers of parental emotion; no doubt they also listen, and glean much explicit and implicit information, when parents talk about their feelings.

Another way in which parents' coaching contributes to ER is via managing what information is given to the child about potentially emotional events. Their attempts to lessen stress may include strategic omission or deemphasis of information. For example, in foretelling the experience of camping in a tent, parents don't mention bears or even raccoons; when talking about learning to swim, they do not describe the "bottomless" feeling at the deep end of the swimming pool. An experience can also be redefined by parents, in a sort of preemptive ER: An injection will only "pinch," or the feeling of a roller-coaster ride makes a person want to say "Wheeeeeeee!" However, some emotional experiences call for greater information in the service of coping, some for less. And some children feel more comfortable with more information, some with less. Parents need to perform a delicate calibration so that this means of ER socialization by discourse does not backfire (Thompson, 1990).

I think that as developmentalists continue to refine the definition of ER, more efforts will be made to substantiate these plausible coaching mechanisms. Some of the most interesting aspects of socialization of emotion may be found in just this area.

## Parents' Reactions to Children's Emotions

Findings on generally positive parenting suggested that parents who are responsive, inductive, warm, and accepting of children's emotional reactions have children who are emotionally well regulated and responsive themselves. The structure and encouragement of autonomy implicit in authoritative parenting require and allow children to make ER attempts.

More specifically, sympathetic parents help children cope effectively with their emotions when they are distressed. Accordingly, these children are less likely to become overaroused. These parents are demonstrating rewarding socialization of emotion. Negative, overbearing parental reactions to children's distress exacerbate child negativity and exemplify punitive socialization of emotion (see Eisenberg, Schaller, et al., 1988; Fabes, Eisenberg, & Miller, 1990; Grolnick et al., 1997). In summary, parental concern over children's need for ER, if it is not punitive, fosters the children's awareness of and attention to their own emotions. In contrast, overly strict sanctions about emotional expressiveness motivate children to hide, not regulate, their emotions.

Several researchers have tested these possibilities even more specifically. Mothers reported on their means of coping with children's negative emotions (Fabes, Eisenberg, & Bernzweig, 1990; Eisenberg & Fabes, 1994; Morales & Bridges, 1997). When they endorsed minimizing/punitive responses (e.g., "I tell my child that he/she is overreacting," or "I tell my child if he/she starts crying then he/she'll have to go to his/her room right away"), their children were more likely to try to escape anger situations, less likely to vent their emotions, and more likely to self-soothe and not to ask their mothers for assistance with ER. Perhaps they had learned only too well the price of showing or becoming involved in emotion.

Mothers who evidenced distress about their children's emotionality (e.g., "I feel upset and uncomfortable because of my child's reaction") had children who were assertive when angry, but did not vent their emotions and showed less intense anger. These children shielded others from their difficult displays of feelings; they wanted to "deal with things" on their own.

Endorsement of problem-focused responses that encouraged constructive action (e.g., "I help my child think of something else to do") were negatively associated with children's anger intensity, but positively associated with coping via escape. These children dealt with emotional issues in ways that defused their feelings, but relatively indirectly.

Emotion-focused reactions on the part of mothers (e.g., "I comfort my child and try to make him/her feel better") were related to children's use of verbal objection as a means of coping with anger, and negatively related to intensity both of anger and venting as a means of coping. The emotional needs of these children were met sufficiently, so that they "used their words" instead of ranting and raving.

Importantly, the associations of most of these reactions to children's emotions with coping responses remained significant even when the contribution of child temperament was statistically controlled for. Mothers' socialization was important over and above children's own emotional reactivity. The patterns that most closely approximate rewarding socialization, emotion- and problem-focused reactions, were most closely allied with children's adaptive coping.

## CHAPTER SUMMARY

Recent advances in our understanding of children's ER are quite hopeful. Much more work remains to be done, however, to examine both developmental change and individual differences in preschoolers' ER. First, definitional bickering needs to cease, and the operationalization of a richer, fuller conception of ER needs to proceed. Second, after the construct is better elucidated, research must continue to include more varied aspects of ER. For example, the work of Eisenberg and Fabes on individual differences in ER includes emotional, cognitive, and behavioral elements, but is not fleshed out equally in each of these areas. At the very least, researchers who focus on only, or even mostly, one aspect of ER should acknowledge that they are doing exactly that—investigating a piece of a larger, more complex picture.

Moreover, several aspects of ER advanced by Cole, Michel, and Teti (1994) also deserve mention here, as well as more empirical consideration. Young children can reduce, generate, or sustain emotional experience by the emotion-related, cognitive, and behavioral means I have already described, but attention should also be paid to the following:

- Their access to a full range of emotions.
- The fluidity and smoothness of their shifts between emotions and the temporal aspects of ER.
- Their conformity with cultural display rules.

- Their integration of mixed emotions (probably best attained after the preschool period; see Chapter 3).
- Their management of emotions *about* emotions.

Operationalization and subsequent investigation of these aspects of the ER of young children, as well as its socialization, are overdue. In addition, more needs to be learned about what children understand about their *own* means of regulating emotion.

In my view, ER represents the pragmatically useful culmination of emotional expressiveness, understanding, and socialization from all the important people in children's lives. As such, it is extremely important to children's success in the social world: it helps them to reach the goals they desire; it helps them to feel better and to feel that they can master their world; it helps them become more socially competent (see Chapter 6); and it helps them become part of their culture (Hyson, 1994).

## NOTES

1. Processing emotional information takes place at either the lower-brain or the cortical level (Izard, 1993a). Of course, only at the cortical level is it "cognitive"; however, instead of adding yet another layer of complexity to this picture, I refer only to cognitive appraisals at the cortical level (within "behavioral" ER), and in passing to the information-processing capacity (and hence "cognitive" ER) at the lower-brain level.
2. As with ER as a whole, there is also a source of confusion in the conceptualization of coping: It is sometimes seen as a process, sometimes as an outcome. The study of ER as a whole and of coping in particular would benefit from more careful thinking, and from both theoretical and empirical distinctions, regarding this issue.
3. Part of the definitional problem is that we researchers in this area are mostly concerned with a child's experience of emotion—an area we admittedly access only peripherally. Partly because of this, we do not as yet separate *at all* the emotional, cognitive, and behavioral aspects of ER in general from those of coping as I have tried to do here. Most of the following examples will refer only to conscious coping.

# Chapter 6

# Contributions of Emotional Expressiveness, Understanding, and Coping to Social Competence

*E*xpression of certain emotions contributes to success in pre-schoolers' social world:

> *Darryl gets mad at Takisha while playing in the dramatic play area, and hits her with a shoe. Takisha acts hurt, Darryl yells, and Takisha yells back. Somehow, through their assertively and clearly conveyed anger, they seem to resolve the conflict.*

Sometimes understanding others' emotions, or one's own, can facilitate interaction.

> *Andy hurts Mohammed, who calls for Ben. Ben then pushes Andy, the instigator, away. Ben's understanding of emotions helps him respond prosocially to his friend.*

> *Three-year-old Miranda understands that Tiffany is only play-acting being angry, because she is the baby in the house corner. Miranda gives*

*Tiffany very solicitous care rather than responding in kind. She even explains to others that this is a posed emotion: "Tiffy's just pretending."*

Sometimes the ability to regulate emotions makes a preschooler a better play partner. As Hyson (1994) has commented, friends' quarrels are sometimes frequent, but peers moderate the intensity of their emotion because they know each other well and want to maintain friendship.

*John really doesn't like it when Pei Lin runs her tricycle right through his sand castle. He's worked so hard! "Hey!" he yells, and he can feel his skin getting all hot and tingly. He's about to hit one of his very best friends. "You shouldn't wreck it!" he shouts. Pei Lin came back over and screechs the trike to a halt. "I'm sorry, John!" They begin to work on building the castle back up together.*

So far I have discussed in much detail the elements of emotional competence—expressiveness, understanding, and ER—as well as their socialization. But why do I deem them so important? It is my general contention, and others', that preschoolers' emotional competence contributes to a crucial developmental task of the period: emerging social competence in the peer world (see, e.g., Lemerise & Gentil, 1992; Walden, Lemerise, & Gentil, 1992). The model put forward in Chapter 1 reserves a central position for the contributions of emotional competence to the daily lives of young children as they interact with others. Children who are able to understand emotion, to express a wide range of emotions in appropriate settings, and to cope with their own and others' emotions are more likely to be seen as competent social partners by both teachers and peers. Joey, the young "pirate" described at the beginning of Chapter 1, is likely to be sought after as a play companion and commended by his teacher because he so readily understands the interplay of his partners' emotions, reacts accordingly, and vividly expresses a variety of predominantly positive feelings himself.

The complex relations between emotional and social competence may be summarized this way (see Walden & Field, 1990): More spontaneously expressive children may be seen as better play partners and more fun to be with. They may also be able to strategically use their expressiveness to obtain social goals. Similarly, children who can understand the emotions experienced by playmates are at an advantage when responding appropriately to others' emotions during play. Because of this asset, they too may be better liked. Finally, children who are more expressive may actually have a better chance of comprehending others' emotional situations because they have "been there."

Accordingly, I now examine the contributions of patterns of emotional expressiveness, understanding of emotions, and coping with one's own and others' emotions to social competence. "Social competence" is broadly defined; it includes the evaluations of peers, parents, or teachers, as well as actual social behaviors relating to initiating and maintaining interaction.

## CONTRIBUTIONS OF EXPRESSIVENESS
## TO SOCIAL COMPETENCE

Emotional expressiveness makes varied and specific contributions to social interaction (Lemerise & Gentil, 1992). In the broadest sense, emotions are useful social signals that can facilitate interaction. When one child smiles at another while approaching their play area, the signal is "I like you. Want to play?"

> In contrast, imagine Antonio's thoughts when Jared screams at him to get away from his Lego construction. It is clear to Antonio and to all onlookers that Jared is very mad and about to attack. Antonio begins to holler, but then, thinking better of this plan, backs off. In a bit, after Jared is calmer, he returns and offers to help build. Jared's emotions offer Antonio immediate, easily processed feedback regarding his own behavior, as well as information about Jared's intentions.

Emotions can also facilitate the understanding of verbal cues. One child's ambiguous statement to another—"Come here"—can take on very different meanings, depending on whether it is accompanied by happiness, sadness, or anger. Such signals provided by emotional expressiveness can influence the beginning of a social interaction, the course of any given interchange, communication within it, and its culmination in friendship or enmity.

A number of investigations of emotional competence, some already described in this book, highlight such relations between preschoolers' observed emotional expressiveness and various indices of social competence. In my work, preschoolers' expressions of specific emotions, as observed during free play in their classrooms, are often associated with ratings of their sociometric likability and/or teachers' evaluations of their friendliness and aggression (Denham, Auerbach-Major, & Blair, 1997; Denham, Blair, Dixon, Schmidt, & DeMulder, 1997; Denham & Burger, 1991; Denham et al., 1990; see also Arsenio et al., 1997; Lemerise, Walden, & Smith, 1997; Walden et al., 1992). Many of these social outcomes depend on whether the emotions expressed during interaction are positive or negative.

## Positive Emotion and Social Competence

Positive affect in particular has great appeal, promoting social interaction and its continuation. People like to be with others who show joy, and young children are no exception to this rule. Even more specifically, emotional positivity helps children initiate and regulate social exchanges (Sroufe, Schork, Motti, Lawroski, & LaFreniere, 1984; Waters, Wippman, & Sroufe, 1979). Duration of cooperation episodes also is longer when there is more happy affect within dyads (Marcus, 1987).

> *Four-year-olds Jamal and LaToya are both playing in the house corner. LaToya is making pretend soup and humming. Jamal approaches and begins to sweep the area with a child-sized broom. Suddenly, LaToya twirls around and smiles, saying, "Want some soup?" Jamal smiles, too. "Yes, I would. Mmmm . . . that's good." LaToya beams at his praise. She then suggests with a grin, "I'm going to work. I need you to vacuum this floor." Jamal does get the toy vacuum, and pretty soon they choose clothes from the dressup box for their roles of executive mom and stay-at-home dad, giggling together. When Jamal drops the plastic vacuum on LaToya's foot, he flashes a tiny smile, as if to say, "I'm sorry. I didn't mean to," so LaToya doesn't get mad. Later, Jamal and LaToya walk to circle time hand in hand, and sit next to each other, still smiling. They are seen together on an everyday basis after this beginning.*

Jamal and LaToya's enjoyment of each other and of their shared activities illustrates how vital positive affect is in the initiation and regulation of social exchanges, in communication during socially directed acts, and in the formation of friendships.

Positive emotion is important in the moment, but it also has a more far-reaching influence. Because patterns of expressiveness are becoming at least somewhat stable during the preschool years, enduring individual differences in expressiveness influence how children view each other, and how teachers see them. Happier children are at an advantage here.

> *Layne is often cheery, with smiles of greeting to teachers and peers alike. She smiles when the teacher announces what song they will be singing in circle time, and the other children join her. She also often expects the other children to follow her lead, and will sternly tell them to do what she wants*

*if they overlook her suggestions. Despite her grouchiness when crossed, they like her, and her teacher sees her as a friendly, though assertive, person.*

Layne's social reputation, based on her positivity, thus becomes established. In particular, preschoolers who evidence better emotion regulation via their balance of happy displays over angry ones are seen as more socially competent: They show more positive attention to their peers' emotions, their peers like them more, and their teachers rate them as more friendly and less aggressive. We have found affective balance to be an  especially important contributor to peers' ratings of boys' likability (Denham, Auerbach-Major, & Blair, 1997; see also Eisenberg et al., 1993).

## Negative Emotion and Social Competence

In contrast, negative affect has aversive and disruptive effects on both ongoing interaction and social information processing about that interaction (Lemerise & Dodge, 1993; Rubin & Clark, 1983; Rubin & Daniels-Byrness, 1983). Like positive emotion, then, negative emotion has effects both at the level of social processes and at the level of social reputation.

> *Three-year-old Carrie is having a very bad day. Her negative emotions, mostly anger, involve her over and over in difficult interactions. She has trouble initiating social exchanges, maintaining them once begun, communicating without fussing, and nurturing friendships. She cries so piteously when her friend Eve uses the "wrong" pretend food in the house corner that a teacher has to comfort her for some time. Then, just after she begins her pretend play again, she yells at Noah when he approaches and unknowingly sits in "her" chair while playing Birthday Party. Sounding quite irritable, she explains, "I have a cold!!" Noah looks thoroughly nonplussed. Later, she screams when she is inadvertently jostled at the play sink. In short, by the end of one 3-hour morning session, neither teachers nor peers want to have anything to do with Carrie. No doubt her screeches are still ringing in their ears.*

Individual differences in anger expression also make a difference in the schemas (and adults, for that matter) children have for each other. Information about enduring anger may reside at the core of people's notions about one another.

> *Connor is often inexplicably grumpy when he comes into the classroom, and he also flares up when crossed. He snarls, "Don't talk to me," and pushes angrily at Jessie when she tries to sits close to him at circle time. Despite the fact that he often gets his way in such interchanges, his*

*classmates rate him as less likable than Layne, and his teachers see him as far more aggressive and definitely less friendly.*

Connor's expressions of unhappiness are more "out of balance" than Layne's, tipped more toward an overall angry demeanor. In line with this example, preschoolers who show larger proportions of negative affect are often seen by teachers and peers alike as troublesome and difficult (Denham, Auerbach-Major, & Blair, 1997; Denham, Blair, et al., 1997; Denham & Burger, 1991; Denham et al., 1990). Their reputations as socially incompetent are becoming stable.

Anger is not the only negative emotion that contributes to the picture of social competence or incompetence. Preschoolers' sadness, whether observed in the classroom or in interaction with their mothers, is related to teachers' ratings of withdrawal and "miserableness," even when child sex and age are statistically controlled for (Denham & Burger, 1991; Denham, Renwick, & Holt, 1991).

*Thomas shows sadness when observed in the preschool, as well as when visiting the laboratory with his mother. His facial demeanor is forlorn, his expressiveness muted. He also often sits alone in school, head down, and is loath to play with others. His social exchange with peers is usually limited to single words. His teachers clearly see him as miserable, isolated, not interacting with others.*

In sum, negativity, when seen as an enduring characteristic of a child, contributes to others' evaluations of the child's abilities to interact with others.

## The Special Role of Empathy

Sympathetic emotional responsiveness is an other important component of emotional competence that supports preschoolers' social competence. Children who respond to the emotional needs of others, sharing positive affect and reacting prosocially to distress, are more likely to succeed in the challenging preschool peer arena (Saarni, 1990; Sroufe et al., 1984).

Specifically, the ability to behave prosocially toward peers—an element of social competence—is linked to empathic emotional responsiveness. Children's facial and gestural sympathy to another's distress is particularly related to their unrequested prosocial behavior. These spontaneously prosocial behaviors constitute a more mature form of prosocial responsiveness associated with social competence, as compared to requested prosocial behavior, which is associated with "wimpiness" (Lennon, Eisenberg, & Carroll, 1986; see also Eisenberg,

McCreath, & Ahn, 1988). Preschoolers who react both empathically and prosocially to their peers' emotions are also seen as more socially competent by both teachers and peers (Denham & Burger, 1991; Denham & Holt, 1993; Marcus, 1980).

It is important, along with observing children and asking important people in their lives how they are doing, to ask the children themselves what's happening. Preschool through grade school children's sympathetic story completions about their own emotional responsiveness to others were related to their actual prosocial behaviors (Chapman, Zahn-Waxler, Cooperman, & Iannotti, 1987). Their observed helping of a kitten, an adult experimenter, and a mother with an infant were also associated with the positive affect that the children attributed to helping itself, and with their guilt over the story protagonist's distress. Thus, the meaning which children attribute to their own emotional arousal when confronted by others' distress, and the accompanying sense of responsibility for the other person's plight, are important affective ingredients of responsiveness to others—itself so important in social relationships. The propensity to cope with others' emotions by expressing sympathy, by feeling guilty, by being pleased about one's helping adds to young children's prosocial development.

## Moderators of the Expressiveness-Social Competence Connection

*Gender*

First, the effects of negative emotion on evaluations of children's social competence may differ by the children's gender. In Eisenberg et al.'s (1993) study, teachers' ratings of boys' negative affect were negatively related to the teachers' ratings of their social skills, as well as to their peer status (but see Denham, Blair, et al., 1997, for opposing results, in which anger and antisocial reactions to peer emotions were negatively related only to ratings of *girls'* social competence[1]). Perhaps these parameters of emotional expressiveness are more vital to boys' social relations because their more intense, more externalizing negativity has a greater impact on their interactions, as well as on teachers' views of them. A clearer picture of these associations would result if the indices of emotion were assessed independently of ratings of social competence, not by the same rater, as was the case in some of Eisenberg and colleagues' analyses.

With respect to the effect of children's sadness during interactions with their mothers (not peers), we also have found a moderating influence of child sex: Boys' sadness with mothers similarly predicted teachers' ratings of their misery in the preschool classroom (Denham,

Renwick, & Holt, 1991). Boys seem to have a special vulnerability to negative affect expressed within the mother–child relationship.

Intensity of boys' versus girls' emotional expressiveness is also likely to be important, although the far-reaching implications of this possibility are by no means clear (Eisenberg et al., 1993; Eisenberg, Fabes, Nyman, Bernzweig, & Pinuelas, 1994; Eisenberg et al., 1995). Intensity of expressiveness may be important in its own right—or only as moderated by gender, and possibly by valence of expressiveness. What is known so far is this: In Eisenberg and colleagues' work, adults rated 5-year-olds' emotional intensity ("This child responds very emotionally to things around him/her"). Mothers' reports of boys' low emotional intensity were associated with teachers' ratings of boys' positive social functioning, but teachers' reports of girls' low emotional intensity were *negatively* related to the teachers' ratings of girls' social competence.

*Context*

Context of expressiveness can also be important; negative emotion does not invariably lead to equally negative evaluations of social competence. Sometimes anger observed in children *positively* predicts teachers' ratings of the children's assertiveness. Thus, expressing prevalent anger can be associated with teachers' perceptions of a sometimes unfriendly and aggressive, sometimes bossy, but socially successful child.

This differentiated view of anger also suggests that the context in which both anger and happiness are expressed is important. Being happy specifically during a conflict is quite a different matter from expressing happiness in general everyday interaction. Having a generally happy demeanor is inviting and an advantage to the development of friendship. But smiling while hitting another child can be seen as very mean, for example; Arsenio et al. (1997) have found that children who show such contextually "misplaced" happiness are less well accepted by their peers. On the other hand, anger during conflict is pretty much expected, and does not predict either peer acceptance or teachers' ratings. But being angry much of the time is a real problem (Arsenio et al., 1997).

## Stability of the Expressiveness–Social Competence Connection

Enduring patterns of emotional expressiveness and equally stable evaluations of social competence during the preschool period (see Denham et al., 1990) hint at the possibility of an increasingly close relation between the two. Many of the predictive relations already reported between expressed emotion and social competence were significant both contemporaneously and over a 1-year period; observations of children's anger in the first year of observation negatively predicted teachers' ratings of friendliness a year later (Denham & Burger, 1991). Withdrawal/misery ratings at Time 2 were also predicted strongly by observed sadness at Time 1; both findings held true when child age and sex were statistically controlled for. Robust cross-time relations such as these underscore the highly salient contribution of young children's emotional expressiveness to evaluations of social competence made by important social partners.

Were these cross-time relations primarily driven by continuity in children's emotional expressiveness—that is, did observers at Time 1 and teachers at Time 2 zero in on the same sorts of evidence? Or did children develop persistent reputations as particularly pleasant or nasty social partners? Either way (or both!), the strong emotional component of interacting with others is already well established by the preschool period, and figures prominently in success in the peer world. Increasingly stable patterns of expressiveness contribute to increasingly stable evaluations of social competence.

## Summary

The expression of emotions is a core component of social interchange. The valence and readability of the emotions that predominate during preschoolers' interactions with others are central to the impression others gain about their skill and attractiveness as play partners. Sadder or angrier children, or those who send mixed, murky emotional messages, are involved in enough problematic exchanges that their developmentally appropriate social relations are compromised. Happier, more empathic children fare much better.

## CONTRIBUTIONS OF UNDERSTANDING OF EMOTIONS TO SOCIAL COMPETENCE

Accurate interpretation of others' emotions provides important information about social situations. The facial expressions of others provide valuable clues to the qualitative meaning of interpersonal exchanges—information that can otherwise be disguised by verbal content. Consider a preschool boy who says, "I am *not* scared of dogs." If he utters these words while chewing on his finger, looking down with a wary expression, a peer understanding his expressive message may feel sympathy that motivates positive, prosocial reactions (Eisenberg, 1986), such as showing the other child how to pet a puppy. Alternatively, a peer who sees this boy tightening his brow and hears him using his gruff tones while making the same statement may take the expedient action of leaving with the puppy and coming back to play later, when the prognosis is more favorable! A third possibility is that accurate interpretation of a peer's subtle cues of pleasure while saying the same thing will allow the preschooler to enter into positive interaction. Children who strategically apply emotion knowledge in highly charged positive and negative situations succeed more often in peer interactions. I would assert that children who have acquired developmentally appropriate emotion knowledge are at a distinct advantage at many crucial moments during play.

## Understanding of Emotions in General

Such understanding of emotions does correlate with a variety of indices of social competence—positive peer status; teachers' ratings of friendliness and aggression; parents' ratings of social competence; children's positive, prosocial reactions to the emotions of others; and even children's own positive perception of their own peer experiences (Denham, 1986; Denham et al., 1990; Denham & Couchoud, 1991; Denham, Auerbach-Major, & Blair, 1997; Denham, Blair, et al., 1997; Field & Walden, 1982; Goldman, Corsini, & de Urioste, 1980; Gnepp, 1989b; Lemerise et al., 1997; Philoppot & Feldman, 1990; Strayer, 1980; Walden et al., 1992). Various components of emotion understanding are represented in these investigators' reports.

In the Field and Walden (1982) study, accurate discriminators of emotional expressions were rated as more extroverted, more popular, and more affectively positive by their teachers.[2] Other investigators have found positive associations between knowledge of basic emotion situations and differing indices of social competence. My colleagues and I have generally utilized an aggregate of comprehension of emotional expressions, both expressive and receptive labels, and situations. Others, such as Gnepp, have examined the relation of more sophisticated, personalized emotion knowledge to social competence. Thus, many aspects of emotion knowledge contribute to various ways of measuring social competence.

The specific types of emotion understanding errors made by young children also predict deficits in social competence. It is easy to envision how particular weaknesses may engender difficulties in the social arena and lead a child to behave in an unpopular way; for example, mistaking a peer's displeasure for pleasure may be particularly dangerous, because the child may continue disliked behaviors. And in fact, we found that confusing happy and sad expressions and situations was negatively related to peer ratings of likability (Denham et al., 1990). Other types of errors, on the other hand, would be more developmentally appropriate, and even logically expected, in the preschool age range: Children at this age often confuse sadness and anger (see also Chapter 3), and such an error was not found to be associated with peer ratings.

## Understanding of One's Own Emotions

Thus, robust and differentiated relations between understanding of emotion and peer status have been found frequently. An investigation by Parke et al. (1992) extended this relation specifically to understanding of one's own emotions. Children were interviewed extensively about their understanding of their own emotions. This understanding was assessed across a range of domains:

- Identification of happiness, sadness, anger, and fear.
- One's experience of each emotion.
- Circumstances leading to one's emotion.
- Expression of one's emotion.
- Behavioral reactions to the display of one's emotion by mother, father, and peer.
- Emotional reactions to the display of one's emotion by mother, father, and peer.

Those who had more positive peer status showed more extensive emotion understanding in every domain except experience of one's emotion (Cassidy, Parke, Butkovsky, & Braungart, 1992; Parke et al., 1992). Moreover, total understanding scores for each separate emotion also predicted peer status as rated by both teachers and peers, especially ratings of overall peer acceptance, shyness, and prosocial behavior. To strengthen these findings, emotion understanding added to the prediction of peer acceptance even when contributions of maternal and paternal expressiveness in both home and laboratory were taken into account (Cassidy et al., 1992). Thus, emotion understanding "mediate[s] the link between family and peer systems" (Parke et al., 1992, p. 123), just as asserted in the model in Figure 1.2 (see Chapter 1).

## Less Global Indices of Understanding of Emotion

There is growing evidence that more discrete elements of emotion knowledge contribute to both particular and molar indices of social competence. For example, use of emotion language—a special demonstration of emotion knowledge—enhances preschoolers' attempts at regulating interpersonal relationships (Kopp, 1989). Knowing how to talk about feelings can help preschoolers convey their needs, get their way, or demonstrate understanding of others. Children learn to use emotion language to influence others' emotional states, as in comforting or asking for comfort, teasing, negotiating, and joking (Dunn, Brown, & Beardsall, 1991). In my work, preschoolers who used more emotion language with their mothers when looking at baby photos, and used more emotion language to explain when their mothers simulated sadness and anger, were rated as more likable by peers up to 9 months later (Denham et al., 1992). Children who can use emotion language in these flexible ways to attain social goals are more skilled with peers and better liked. Sometimes emotion language is central to social success:

> *Todd has already been branded by both his day care providers and his classmates as a difficult guy to be around. After learning a good deal of emotion language from one teacher, though, he is heard taking part in a very heated discussion, replete with feeling terms, negotiating an object struggle with a friend. The boys' smiles at the end of their argument testify to the power of emotion language to contribute to Todd's newfound social success.*

Understanding of family emotion is also a special form of emotion knowledge. Unlike the quantitative measures of emotion knowledge that predict peer status and teacher-rated social competence, however, more qualitative parameters of children's conceptions of their parents' emotions are the important predictors. Children who more frequently depicted parents as comforting or as matching their positive emotions were seen by teachers as more skilled with peers, more cooperative, and more empathic (Denham, 1997). In contrast, children who more frequently depicted parents as matching negative emotions were seen as less cooperative. Children who more frequently depicted their parents as discussing emotions were seen as more empathic. These coherent and complete conceptions about family emotion predicted aspects of social competence. They also paralleled affect sharing and distress relief, which are important components of young children's internal working models of emotional security (Denham, 1997; Thompson, 1990).

Furthermore, children who were able to describe the causes, typical expression, and resolution of their parents' emotions were rated as more socially competent overall (Denham, 1996a). Hence, preschoolers' interpretations of family emotions are essential reflections of their notions about emotional reality. Children with richer, more complete, but also more emotionally secure conceptions of their families' affective environment are more able to succeed with their friends and school routine.

Finally, one last specific aspect of emotion knowledge—knowledge of display rules—is associated with later social competence (Jones et al., in press). Knowing when and when not to show emotions is intimately tied to the success of ongoing social interaction. Thus it is not surprising that those preschoolers who are better at this developmentally advanced skill are seen as more socially adept.

## Less Global Indices of Social Competence

Emotion understanding is also related to more particular components of social competence. In one study, one particular aspect of emotion understanding contributed to young children's responsiveness to the emotional needs of others: Emotional role taking, the ability to "be open to and recognize the unique cues generated by the individual in a particular situation," predicted preschoolers' caregiving toward their younger siblings during a modified 4-minute Strange Situation (Garner, Jones, & Palmer, 1994, p. 910). In another study, both emotion situation knowledge and emotional role taking, which permit children to understand both unequivocal and more equivocal situational sources of emotion, contributed to preschoolers' ability to remain positive in a disappointing circumstance (Garner & Power, 1996). These aspects of emotion understanding also predicted lower levels of aggression in Arsenio et al.'s (1997) investigation.

Moral development may be facilitated by emotion understanding as well. Dunn, Brown, and Maguire (1995) first administered my puppet measure of understanding of emotions when children were 40 months old, and then Gordis et al.'s (1989; see also Chapter 3) measure of understanding of ambivalent emotions when the children entered kindergarten. All children responded to three separate lines of questioning. First, they were explicitly told that a story protagonist felt two emotions at the same time, in situations such as receiving a present and not being allowed to open it, or anticipating the last day of school. They justified the two feelings for each story. In the second part, they were told stories and asked to tell how the protagonist felt; in the third part, they were asked to tell a story of a time they had felt two different feelings at the same time themselves. Kindergarten children and first-grade children also responded to a narrative measure of feelings about moral transgressions, such as cheating: "How would you feel?

Why? What would you feel if no one found out (and why)? What will happen next?"

Young children's early understanding of emotion buttressed their moral sensibility. Their ability to identify emotional expressions and situations, as indexed by the puppet measure administered earlier in the preschool period, was related to a more empathic moral orientation and more reparative story completions in kindergarten. Those who scored higher in kindergarten on understanding of emotional ambivalence also showed more empathic moral orientation and more intense discomfort on the story completion measure in first grade. So developmentally appropriate understanding of emotion forms a foundation for young children's morality, over and above intelligence and verbal ability.

Discovering these linkages between emotion understanding and moral thinking is very exciting. Such findings support Arsenio and Lover's (1995) model of sociomoral development: Children witness emotions, think about emotion–event links, and use these emotion-related cognitions to contribute to their moral reasoning and behavior. Given the success of these efforts, more research should be undertaken to examine the association of important subareas of social competence and peer acceptance with understanding of emotion.

## Summary

In the last decade, more researchers, instead of studying only the normative social-cognitive attainment of the toddler-to-preschool period, have begun to entertain the notion that young children exhibit individual differences in the understanding of emotions. Clearly, exploring these individual differences has shown that they are contributors to social competence as reported by a wide range of raters.

## CONTRIBUTIONS OF EMOTION REGULATION TO SOCIAL COMPETENCE

Expressiveness itself is, as shown above, an important part of skilled social interaction and a predictor of the assessments made by people in the child's social world. But sometimes emotions need to be regulated (see Chapter 5). So not only is the relative profile of the child's expression of positive and negative emotions important; the child's ability to deal with these emotions, or ER, is also vital.

Unfortunately, there is as yet little research specifically on the relation of ER to social competence. Most such research has been performed by Eisenberg et al. (1993, 1994, 1995). Teachers and mothers captured children's coping techniques in two ways. First, they rated the likelihood that each child would ever engage in a number of coping techniques—instrumental coping, crying to elicit help, instrumental aggression, avoidance, distraction, venting, emotional aggression, cognitive restructuring, seeking emotional support, cognitive avoidance, instrumental intervention, seeking instrumental support, and denial. They also rated the child's likelihood of coping in these ways in specific everyday conflict scenarios. These coping scales were finally collapsed into aggregates of constructive coping and acting out versus avoidance. Second, the children's intensity of emotion was rated by teachers, and their intensity of anger was observed as an index of their ability to modulate their feelings.

Teachers' ratings of boys' constructive coping were positively related to social competence, as rated by both aides and teachers, and to sociometric status (see also Denham, Auerbach-Major, & Blair, 1997, for findings not differentiated by sex). Mothers' reports of boys' coping by seeking social support were associated with boys' positive social functioning. A picture emerges, then, of the socially competent boys using a flexible assortment of coping methods to deal with strong feelings that erupted during their interactions with each other. These relations held true both contemporaneously and over a 2-year period. Being passive or avoidant in emotional situations seemed to be a particularly ineffective, debilitating means of coping for boys: Teachers saw these boys as actually showing *more* anger 1 year later (Denham, Blair, et al., 1997).

In contrast, girls' rated social skills were positively related to avoidant coping, but no other significant relations were reported (again, see Denham, Auerbach-Major, & Blair, 1997, and Denham, Blair, et al., 1997, for findings not differentiated by sex). So, girls seen as socially competent were those who tended to deal less actively with difficult situations. It is likely that girls in general are already socialized into more uniformly "nice," controlled, and culturally approved competent social behavior. For them, the important determinants of sociometric preference and being seen as competent by their teachers may be less determined by this aspect of emotional competence, and more so by other facets of their social interaction and personality (e.g., their cooperativeness).

These findings show that the ability to cope with emotions makes important contributions to social competence. However, one criticism of Eisenberg and colleagues' work is that core findings centered on teachers' ratings of both coping and social competence. Hence, an alternative interpretation is that shared method variance accounts for the association between coping and social competence. To avert such alternative explanations, and to extend their earlier findings, Eisenberg et al. (1994) evaluated the associations between ratings of the 5-year-olds' social competence and *observed* means of dealing with their own anger. Peer acceptance and teacher ratings of social competence were related to young children's observed use of verbal objections when angry, a relatively socially competent tactic, even when contributions of sex and age were statistically controlled for.

Again, some intriguing findings were gender-specific. For girls, observed venting when angry was negatively related to teacher ratings of social competence, whereas use of escape tactics was positively related. The socially competent preschool girls again used more avoidant coping tactics. In contrast, boys' social competence was not related to emotion-regulatory coping.

Overall, these adult informants considered children's means of coping in emotion-filled social conflict situations relatively more important than their intensity of emotional expressiveness in predicting their social skills. But as our means of pinpointing dimensions of expressiveness, its regulation, and coping become more clearly specified and more sharply differentiated, we may find that preschoolers who demonstrate *under*regulated high-intensity emotions look very different socially from those few whose emotions are highly intense but already well regulated (Eisenberg et al., 1993, 1996).

In short, the research findings beginning to trickle into the literature suggest that young children's constructive means of coping with strong emotions are associated with adults' views of their social functioning, especially for boys. Although these important investigations need to proceed, and gender-specific pictures especially need to be clarified, caregivers should be encouraged in their attempts to scaffold preschoolers' efforts to cope with emotions.

## DIRECT CONTRIBUTIONS OF PARENTS' EMOTION-RELATED SOCIALIZATION TO SOCIAL COMPETENCE

The model I have put forward in this volume emphasizes that socialization of emotion affects social competence indirectly via the mediation of children's emotional competence. But, of course, it is possible that the reassuring constellation of parenting strategies I have called "rewarding socialization of emotion" makes a direct contribution to elements of young children's social competence. So, in their recent consideration of the influence of parent–child interaction on children's competence in the peer group, some researchers have examined the direct effects of emotion socialization techniques.

In one line of research, investigators have focused on parents' expressiveness as measured by specific emotions observed during interaction with their children. Not only should the children's expression of positive and negative emotion contribute to children's peer acceptance, but parents' expression of positive and negative emotion may also make a direct contribution (Butkovsky, 1991), presumably through modeling of socially appropriate functioning in emotional situations.

In Butkovsky's study, mother–child and father–child dyads played a ball-toss game and a ring-toss game. Each child played four times, but the game was rigged: the child won the first and fourth trials, but lost the middle two trials. Parents were given vague instructions requiring them to participate relatively passively in the experience. Nonetheless, their peak positive affect was associated with children's peer acceptance, especially for fathers and girls. Appropriateness of affect was related to children's peer acceptance, especially for sons and mothers. Thus, dimensions of parents' emotional competence—their positive and appropriate expressiveness—predicted their children's likability.

In another effort to study the direct contribution of family emotions to peer relations, Carson and Parke (1996) also utilized a game-playing context. Children aged 4 and 5, who had previously been identified as popular or rejected, and their parents played a "hand game." The object was for the first person to reach out and grab the other's hands before that person pulled them away. Popular and rejected preschoolers and their parents displayed different patterns of facial, vocal, and gestural emotion. Parents of rejected children showed more anger and more neutrality, whereas those of popular children gave more affect-laden guidance and apologized more.

Other researchers have focused on the overall family affective environment in searching for direct links between family and peer systems. Kindergartners who varied in popularity were observed with their parents during dinner, and parents reported on emotional expressiveness in their families (Boyum & Parke, 1995). Results in this study were father-specific: Those who self-reported higher levels of expressiveness also showed more positive affect and less negative affect in the home. Fathers who reported more positive expressiveness overall and showed less negative affect during dinner also had more popular children. So both specific expressed emotions and the overall affective environment, particularly for fathers (who have been too often ignored in socialization of emotion research), are important to young children's social competence.

Maternal and paternal expressiveness in the home and paternal emotions in a laboratory ring-toss game similarly predicted peer acceptance in yet another study (Cassidy et al., 1992). An important addition to the general findings noted above was that the children's overall understanding of emotions influenced this link between parental emotion and social competence. That is, statistically controlling for emotion understanding in the prediction of peer status lessened the predictive strength of parental emotion. Although the total mediation effect predicted in Figure 1.2 was not upheld, the child's emotion understanding buffered too-little or too-intense family emotion.

Contingent reactions to children's emotions also directly predict social competence. Encouragement and support for children's emotions help them to express emotion acceptably and provide children with ways to deal with emotions *in the peer group*, which then influence evaluations of social competence. Punitive socialization of emotion increases arousal and undermines the performance of socially competent interacting. In my own work, parents' self-reported and observed positive and negative emotions and positive reactions to child emotions predicted teacher-rated social competence even after children's negative emotions in preschool and antisocial reactions to paternal emotions were statistically controlled for (Denham, Mitchell-Copeland, et al., 1994, 1997). This set of findings suggests that not only parental expressiveness, but also parents' accepting reactions to their children's emotions, predict social competence even when children's own emotional competence is already accounted for. Furthermore, older siblings' rewarding socialization—their positive responsiveness, lack of ignoring, and prosocial reactions to their younger siblings' emotions—predicts their younger brothers' and sisters' own positive reactions to peer emotions and teacher-rated social competence (Sawyer, 1996).

More molar patterns of parent–child emotional contingency also directly predict social competence. In the Carson and Parke (1996) study, different sequences of child–parent emotions were revealed for popular and rejected children playing with same-sex parents. Rejected boys playing with fathers and popular girls playing with mothers showed more negative affect reciprocity than their same-sex, opposite-sociometric-status counterparts. The pattern for popular daughters and mothers is a bit difficult to explain (except to mothers of daughters!), but Carson and Parke noted that there were intensity differences in the negative affect of the two dyad types. Popular girls, they reasoned, are learning assertion, as opposed to the aggression rejected sons learn in interactions with their fathers.

Long-term outcomes have been reported by Hooven, Katz, and Gottman (1994). These researchers found that rewarding socializers of emotion had children who not only got along better with them, but were also better at handling their own emotions, more popular, more socially competent, and even more physiologically relaxed. Amazingly, they also had higher mathematics and reading achievement scores by third grade. My interpretation of these findings is that emotional competence developed early gave these children a head start on the social aspects of schooling, so that they could focus on academics. As Goleman (1995) asserts, "the payoff for children whose parents are [rewarding socializers] is a surprising—almost astounding—range of advantages across, and beyond, the spectrum of emotional intelligence" (p. 192). In sum, these rewarding socialization techniques promote the integrated emotional organization of personality.

Thus it is clear that socialization of emotion techniques *may* directly influence social competence, without mediation by emotional competence (direct contributions of various elements of parental coaching, such as their emotion language, have not yet been demonstrated). However, in the majority of these studies (with the exception of those by Cassidy and colleagues and by our group), there is no way of knowing whether emotional competence mediated the effects of parental socialization of emotion. Elements of emotional competence in the preschool were not tested or rated.

But both direct and indirect mediated effects are possible, and these should continue to be explored. More explicit attention also should be given to *why* a parent's socialization of emotion should directly predict evaluation of another person's (the child's) social competence. Finally, an interactive approach might be profitable— examining whether emotionally competent children of rewarding socializers are at least risk for social competence problems (or vice versa; see Auerbach-Major, Kochanoff, & Queenan, 1997, for findings supportive of this proposition).

## CHAPTER SUMMARY

Recent explorations confirm that the central elements of preschool emotional competence posited here are indeed related to success in the preschool/day care environment. Children who are relatively positively expressive and clear in their expressiveness, who know how to cope with negative emotions when these do occur, and who understand their own and others' emotions are liked by peers and considered friendly, cooperative, assertive, prosocial, and nonaggressive by their teachers and independent observers. Because early peer experience is pivotal to later social and cognitive attainments, even more attention should be paid to these issues. Careful multisetting, multimethod work needs to continue, and more specific areas of social competence need to be considered, as Dunn et al. (1995) have begun to do in their study of moral sensibility and understanding of emotion. Finally, the full direct and indirect models of parental contribution to emotional and social competence must be more clearly defined.

## NOTES

1. Teachers may *expect* boys to be more angry and aggressive, and their ratings of such behaviors may be based more on reputation or other factors than on direct observation. Conversely, when they do witness anger and antisocial reactions to peer emotions in girls, they may factor these into their social competence ratings more directly.
2. *Sending* clear emotional messages is also important during peer interaction. Field and Walden (1982) also tested young children's production of facial expression of emotions under "posed" and "unposed" conditions (see Chapter 2). Children who were accurate producers of emotions were rated by their teachers as more affectively positive, popular, and extroverted.

## ❧ Chapter 7

# Disruptions in the Development of Emotional Competence and Interventions to Ameliorate Them

$M$any factors in children or their environment can compromise their developing emotional competence. Some preschoolers' emotional competence is at risk because of intrapersonal factors.

*Jeff has been diagnosed with pervasive developmental disorder. He appears rather emotionally flat most of the time, but he sometimes erupts in contextually confusing laughter or rage. He seems oblivious to the emotional output of his developmentally delayed and nondelayed classmates.*

Other preschoolers' emotional competence is at risk because of interpersonal factors.

*Carla's mother suffers from major depressive disorder. When they are together–if she is awake–she is loving, but in a clingy, whining way that makes her, not 2½-year-old Carla, seem the "baby." She talks with great exhaustion about how to just make it through the day, and her monologue is laced with references to her need for Carla to be a "good girl." No wonder Carla is rather unemotional but very, very compliant when observed in her preschool class. Her play is restricted, but when other children cry hard, she looks pained and often intervenes in some way. Nonetheless, she performs less well than expected for her age on measures of emotion understanding.*

The development of preschoolers' emotional expressiveness, understanding of emotions, and regulation of emotions does not always go smoothly. Thus, in this chapter I address three major issues. First, I detail disturbances of emotional competence that are consonant with conditions existing within the child; those in which environmental contributors are prominent; and, finally, those with mixed contributors—partly intra- and partly interpersonal. Next, I outline and evaluate major means of identifying and assessing such deficits. Finally, I discuss specific interventions that can be used to ameliorate disruptions in the development of emotional competence.

## BIOLOGICAL CONTRIBUTIONS TO DISRUPTIONS IN EMOTIONAL COMPETENCE

Two exemplary cases of biological contributions to emotional competence deficits are autism and Down syndrome. Autism is characterized by extensive deficits in both cognitive and social-emotional domains. Specific features of autistic disorder include the following: lack of awareness of the feelings of others, little or no facial expressiveness for communication, distress over trivial changes in the environment, and abnormal comfort seeking under distress (see also Cole, Michel, & Teti, 1994). Thus autistic children show both qualitatively and quantitatively impoverished indicators of emotional competence. An autistic child's lack of social responsiveness is reflected in lack of expressiveness, with autism's characteristic cognitive and social-emotional deficits accompanied by deficits in understanding and regulation of emotions.

In contrast, the emotional competence deficits associated with Down syndrome are more clearly due to cognitive/intellectual delay, especially in the areas of emotion understanding and ER. Furthermore, Down syndrome is accompanied by hypotonicity of the facial muscles which causes qualitative differences in children's patterns of emotional expressiveness.

## Autistic Children and Emotional Competence

Regarding emotional expressiveness, autistic preschoolers display happy, sad, angry, and neutral facial expressions at a frequency similar to that of age-matched normal children. But they are more likely to make these displays during contextually incongruent situations (McGee, Feldman, & Chernin, 1991). This intriguing finding reminds us that the expression of various emotions may be biologically based— *all* children show emotions. However, autistic children's deficits in joint attention and sensory integration make it difficult for them to learn *when* to show specific emotions. They may be unable to receive and assimilate socialization messages about what emotions to show in varying situations.

So autistic children show emotions, but in inappropriate contexts. There is evidence that they smile less during peer interaction, and that in such settings they are less likely than nondelayed children to coordinate their emotional displays with eye contact (Lord & Magill-Evans, 1995). They also show more incongruous blends of emotions (e.g., joy and sadness; Yirmiya, Kasari, Sigman, & Mundy, 1989). Furthermore, autistic children do not show positive affect in typical situations, such as during interaction with their mothers or with peers (Dawson, Hill, Spencer, Galpert, & Watson, 1990; Mundy, Kasari, & Sigman, 1992; Snow, Hertzig, & Shapiro, 1987). Regarding the expression of self-conscious emotions, children with autism smile when they complete difficult tasks such as puzzles, but do not look up to others or draw attention to their accomplishments (Kasari, Sigman, Baumgartner, & Stipek, 1993).

Taken together, these findings show that the expressiveness of autistic children is distinguished by qualitatively, not quantitatively, important social differences. As Kasari and Sigman (1996, p. 115) have stated, "A brief expression that appears odd and does not fit the tone of [an] interaction may significantly disrupt the flow of the interaction." Moreover, these socially important differences are lasting: There seems to be significant stability in autistic children's emotional responses over a 5-year period (Dissanayake, Sigman, & Kasari, 1996).

Causal understanding of emotional situations, desires, and beliefs was tested in autistic children (Baron-Cohen, 1991). They did not differ from developmentally disabled, nonautistic children in their understanding of unequivocal situations that cause emotions (e.g., going to the zoo makes everyone happy) or of the desires associated with the experience of emotions (e.g., when a boy gets what he wants, he is happy). Both groups performed less well than nondiagnosed children. In contrast, autistic children demonstrated specific and severe deficits in comprehension of emotion caused by beliefs (e.g., a girl is sad because she believes she is about to lose her toy forever when her brother takes it). Thus, belief—a specific element of autistic children's "theory of mind"—was particularly difficult for them to utilize, especially in conjunction with emotional information.[1]

Regarding autistic children's ER (their ability to cope with emotions), these children's attention and behavioral and emotional reactions to adult displays of pain and fear differed from those of nonautistic children in one study (Sigman, Kasari, Kwon, & Yirmiya, 1992). They spent significantly *less* time looking at a distressed or fearful adult than did matched groups of children with either typical development, or developmental delay. The autistic children showed a different pattern—a different notion of what was important—in situations where an adult injured himself or herself or was accosted by a strange robot. They looked at, for example, the pounding toys that resulted in the adult's self-injury. Although they also were rated as less concerned than the other two groups, the autistic children did seem influenced by the adult's demonstration of fear. Their latency to approach the robot was greater and their play with it less extensive than when fear was not displayed, even though they did not attend visually to the adult's display of fear. Thus, the children somehow made use of emotional information to guide their own behavior in the service of coping, but in a typically detached way.

In summary, the *social* side of emotional competence—for instance, displaying emotions in "appropriate" situations, or attending to others' emotions in order to respond socially—is lacking or delayed in children with this pervasive developmental disability.[2]

## Down Syndrome Children and Emotional Competence

In some ways, Down syndrome children are very similar to their normally developing counterparts; in others, they are quite different. Like their nondelayed counterparts, Down syndrome children show stable expressive styles in the emotion-related components of temperament (although such stability is greater for nondisabled children; Vaughn et al., 1993). In contrast, there are mean differences in these stable attributes of emotionality across groups: Down syndrome children, compared with nondelayed children, are generally hard to arouse emotionally and rather placid. Once aroused, they have more difficulty with ER. Some of this apparent composure is undoubtedly due to the poor muscle tone common to this syndrome; these children show briefer, less intense expressions that do not involve the entire face (Kasari, Mundy, Yirmiya, & Sigman, 1990).

Nonetheless, these are rather subtle differences, which functionally may be relatively unimportant. Furthermore, like nondiagnosed children, Down syndrome children show pride—positive affect expression and social orientation at task completion (Hughes & Kasari, 1995). On some dimensions, then, expressive differences are not large between Down syndrome and nondisabled children; in these areas, the development of expressiveness follows a common path in the two groups. Down syndrome children do communicate their feelings and have their own unique "emotional styles."

In contrast, emotion understanding is often compromised in developmentally handicapped children, including those with Down syndrome. In one study, both developmentally handicapped and autistic children performed more poorly than mental-age-matched preschoolers on encoding and decoding skills—imitating and labeling another person's emotions. The developmentally handicapped children's relative strength was in imitating (the "posed" expressiveness I have discussed in Chapter 2), whereas that of the autistic children was in labeling emotions (Hertzig, Snow, & Sherman, 1989). So autistic children have trouble *expressing* emotions, whereas Down syndrome children have trouble *comprehending* them.

But are these deficits in understanding emotions, like the expressive deficits of autistic children, qualitative and pervasive? Or are they merely quantitative? Kasari, Hughes, and Freeman (1994) examined Down syndrome children's understanding of emotion with my puppet measure. On this measure, which requires almost no verbalization, 4- to 6-year-old Down syndrome children performed as well as developmental-age-matched nondisabled children. Thus, their understanding of emotion was understandably developmentally delayed, but it showed only one actual anomaly: Most of the Down syndrome children's errors were in saying the puppet was happy when it was not (a positive bias).

So Down syndrome children's deficits in understanding of emotions are quantitative, not qualitative. Taken together, these often complex results suggest that Down syndrome children are sometimes, but not always, different from nondisabled children in certain aspects of both expressiveness and understanding of emotion—two components of emotional competence. Their ER, however, has not been adequately tested. Kasari, Mundy, and Sigman (1990) examined Down syndrome children's reactions to an adult examiner when she pretended to hurt her finger and cry. Unlike more typically developing children, Down syndrome children showed more neutral and negative expressions, rather than interest or quizzical expressions. The Down syndrome children looked upset themselves more often than they looked as if they were trying to "figure out" the situation. Moreover, they looked for a long time almost as if they were having difficulty understanding what was happening—failing to make connections between the event and the emotions. These reactions are similar to those of younger children, as might be expected (Cummings, 1987; see Chapter 5).

Overall, it is clear that conditions arising mainly "within" children, such as autism and Down syndrome, can contribute to deficits in young children's emotional competence. There are not merely unarticulated delays in all areas, however; delays for each group fit logically with the nature of their diagnoses. Despite what is known so far, more research is needed to give a more complete picture of all the components of emotional competence in autistic and Down syndrome children.

## ENVIRONMENTAL CONTRIBUTIONS TO DISRUPTIONS IN EMOTIONAL COMPETENCE

The emphasis I place on socialization of emotion points to the importance of socializers', especially parents', potentially detrimental contributions to young children's delays in emotional competence. One foremost exemplar of the environmental disruption of emotional competence development is child maltreatment; another is parental affective disturbance. In families where either of these problems exist, the emotion socialization environment is affectively, if not physically, punishing and unpredictable. Aberrant modeling of emotional displays, coaching about emotions, and contingent reactions to children's emotions are all quite possible in such settings. I consider these contributors to deficits in young children's emotional competence in turn.

### Maltreatment and Emotional Competence

First, young children's expression and experience of emotion are altered substantially by unpredictable, harsh treatment from the very persons who are also their caregivers. Two recent investigations of maltreated children's behavioral and emotional self-regulation suggest that maltreatment exerts a far-ranging, deleterious effect on children's profile of expressiveness (Rogosch, Cicchetti, & Aber, 1995; Shields, Cicchetti, & Ryan, 1994). Maltreated children as young as 2 years old exhibit more anger, and more situationally inappropriate, nonadaptively intense, inflexible emotions, when compared to nonmaltreated children (Erickson, Egeland, & Pianta, 1989; Shields et al., 1994). Not surprisingly, they express fear when hurt by a peer, rather than more appropriate "righteous anger." They are also more emotionally labile, and they demonstrate depression, anxiety, and shame (Alessandri & Lewis, 1996; Rogosch et al., 1995; Toth, Manly, & Cicchetti, 1992). Finally, maltreated children's expressive patterns are less readable for their social partners (see Camras, Ribordy, & Hill, 1988).

Nonempathic reactions to others' emotions are well documented for toddlers living in circumstances of abuse and neglect. Instead of expressing empathy or sympathy, abused toddlers were found to demonstrate more "abusive" emotional patterns in response to peers' distress, including intense anger or fear (Main & George, 1985; see also George & Main, 1979). In these studies, not one abused toddler showed concern in response to a peer's distress. Toddlers from families where there was stress, but no abuse, showed no such anomalous behavior; instead, they showed interest, concern, empathy, or sadness, as would be expected developmentally.

Maltreated preschoolers show similar, perhaps even more pervasive distortions in their emotional expressiveness contingent upon peers' emotions. Howes and Eldredge (1985) observed abused, neglected, and nonmaltreated preschoolers in structured and free-play settings; groups were matched on developmental status, age, height, weight, demographic factors, and time in day care (see also Klimes-Dougan & Kistner, 1990). These observations, in contrast to those of toddlers, extended to the preschoolers' reactions not only to peers' distress, but also to their anger and happiness.

Maltreated preschoolers, like toddlers, respond to peers' distress inappropriately, with angry aggression or sad withdrawal. These deficits in maltreated preschoolers' empathy even extend to self-report procedures (Straker & Jacobson, 1981). Nonmaltreated children offer distressed peers their empathy. When faced with angry, aggressive peers, maltreated preschoolers respond in kind; in contrast, nonmaltreated children usually cry. Only maltreated children routinely resist peers' affectively positive overtures during play.

Overall, then, maltreated toddlers' and preschoolers' reactions to others' emotions are atypical—alternately unconcerned and punitive. In peer settings, maltreated youngsters are relatively unable to share others' positive affect, relieve their distress, or defuse their anger. When opportunities for prosocial emotional responsiveness arise during interaction with peers, then, young maltreated children do not rise to the occasion.

The life situation of maltreated children elicits negative emotions and promotes the development of these nonoptimal expressiveness patterns. It is easy to see how expecting anger from others and not having distress relieved could disrupt young children's own emotionality. Through their own difficult circumstances, these children feel justifiable fear when confronted with *anyone's* anger, see a need for self-defense where none exists, consider anger an automatic response to many social challenges, and learn nonempathic responses to others' distress. Understandably, they are easily overwhelmed by common emotional experiences, and they project their own experience onto the canvas of any emotional topic (Sachs-Alter, 1993). The emotional expression and experience of maltreated children thus become difficult to tolerate, from both their own and other people's perspectives. This set of expressive patterns can be seen not only as an outcome of a maltreatment history, but as a contributor to continued difficulty with the maltreating parents, other caregivers, and peers.

The principle of functional adaptation, in which seemingly maladaptive behavior patterns develop in children and persist over time (Malatesta, 1990), also helps explain these expressiveness patterns. Returning to a functional analysis of emotions shows the expressiveness of maltreated preschoolers in a different light: Their developing expressive patterns meet the unique goals emerging from their life circumstances. "The fear reactions of [maltreated] children, with the submissive content that fear postures convey, may help [maltreating mothers] keep hostile impulses in check" (Malatesta, 1990, p. 35). Furthermore, it is not surprising that these children show frequent anger—an emotion mobilized to overcome obstructions to goals and to notify social partners of one's frustration. Positive affect promotes potentially dangerous social bonding, so that its relative lack makes sense.

The development of understanding of emotion is also hindered in maltreated children. In comparisons of maltreated and nonmaltreated children, nonmaltreated 4- and 5-year-olds were better able to recognize both "pure" and "masked" emotions, such as happiness, sadness, anger, fear, surprise, and disgust, when compared to maltreated children matched on demographics and intelligence (Camras et al., 1988, 1990; During & McMahon, 1991). Moreover, maltreated children were less able to demonstrate the more complex emotion understanding skills discussed in Chapter 3: processing multiple pieces of conflicting facial and situational emotional information, using personalized information, and integrating complex emotion messages (Sachs-Alter, 1993).

Unfortunately, the environmental source of this disruption in emotional competence was not uncovered in Camras et al.'s investigations, because maltreating and nonmaltreating mothers did not differ in facial expressions. That is, both groups of mothers were similar in the expression and modeling of their own emotions, *when observed.* Theoretically, then, both groups could foster equivalent emotion understanding by allowing their children to observe similar expression–situation linkages.

What then explains the groups' differences in emotion understanding? Because developmental outcomes depend not only on the nature of socialization, but also on a child's processing of such socialization, Camras et al. have theorized that maltreated children may not make optimal use of their similar affective experiences with parents. Young maltreated children experience maternal emotion as so aversive, or as such a pointed signal of upcoming peril, that they cope by not attending or by not processing emotional information when they do attend. This strategy makes good intuitive sense: In a similar vein, one 3-year-old daughter of a bipolar mother, when witnessing our puppet's expressions of anger, turned her back and emphatically stated, "I will play when her is not mad no more."

Another plausible explanation is that maltreating mothers differ in their expressiveness only during rarely observed but highly charged emotional situations—that is, when their children misbehave. The intensity of maternal anger during episodes of maltreatment may poignantly differentiate maltreating mothers from nonmaltreating ones; such high-intensity negative emotion may spark the postulated process of children's inattention to that emotion and to emotions in general. So maltreating mothers may not differ from nonmaltreating mothers in their overall expressive profile, their modeling of expressiveness. Or they may differ in very infrequent but, sadly, extremely salient events.

Maltreating mothers clearly differ in another important area of socialization of emotion—in their reactions to their children's emotions, particularly in deliberate expressions produced to comment on their children's emotions. Nonmaltreating mothers show negative expressions to stress the seriousness of their instructions to children, but not in response to the children specifically. In contrast, maltreating mothers are more punitive in their specific reactions to children's emotions (Sachs-Alter, 1989). They are unlikely to show positive expressions in response to their children's positive affect, and are likely to show negative expressions in a wide range of child-centered situations. These reactions of constant negativity and dissatisfaction encourage the children to shut down regarding experiencing (and thus understanding) emotions altogether.

Maltreating mothers may also show skewed or idiosyncratic reactions to their children's emotions, so that the children themselves learn nonnormative conceptions of emotion. They may exhibit more maladaptive coaching about emotions, focusing on anger or giving mixed or garbled messages about emotions. All of these possibilities could be partly explanatory of Camras and colleagues' results, and should be sensitively tested in further research.

Another aspect of young children's understanding of emotions, emotion language, is adversely affected by maltreatment. Maltreated toddlers use fewer internal state words as early as 30 months of age, especially those referring to negative emotion (Beeghly & Cicchetti, 1994). In the service of maintaining their own equilibrium, they suppress reference to the intense negative emotions they witness. Furthermore, even when they do talk about emotion, they less often discuss their mothers' internal states or refer back to them after their occurrence. These deficiencies in ongoing conversation make sense, given the hostile affective environment of these youngsters.

The importance of these deficits in emotion understanding cannot be underestimated. Early inability to understand negative emotions can mediate both the relation of maltreatment on later dysregulated behavior in a peer setting, and the effect of maltreatment on later rejection by peers (Rogosch et al., 1995). In other words, children who are maltreated experience a delay in their early understanding of negative emotions, and this deficit predicts later maladaptive behavior with peers and consequent rejection. The pathway from emotional to social competence is compromised for these children.

In regard to ER, maltreated children's life experiences make it logical to assume that they will also find it difficult to cope with the contagion of others' anger. So far, however, research on this component of emotional competence involves only older maltreated children. School-age maltreated children do not habituate to interadult hostility involving their mothers (Cummings, Hennessy, Rabideau, & Cicchetti, 1994). In fact, the chronic, intense, unresolved conflict inherent in a maltreating environment fosters their emotional arousal and aggression. When an angry experimenter confronts their mothers, maltreated children are more likely than nonmaltreated children to be angry or aggressive themselves. They are also more likely to show concern in the form of attempts to help, comfort, or intervene for their mothers.

It would be interesting to scale down this research with younger participants. For example, would maltreated preschoolers also try to nurture their mothers, showing empathy toward them that they do not exhibit with peers? My guess is that they would. When reacting to the distress of a similar-status peer, a maltreated child probably quickly resorts to an offensive, goal-oriented posture: To ignore the other's distress and continue playing, or to show aggression in response, means getting what the child wants. But reactions to a potentially maltreating mother probably serve a self-protective, defensive function: To take care of the mother means not getting hurt physically or emotionally.

Thus, young children seem to be at definite risk for emotional competence deficits in several areas when they experience maltreatment. In particular, they show less typical patterns of understanding emotions and empathic responsiveness to the emotions of others. These two major deficit areas make much sense when we reflect on the likely life experience of the young maltreated child. Exposure to a parent's overwhelming negative emotion, which is accompanied by equally negative behavior, can alter the child's understanding of emotion via the routes suggested. Furthermore, when the child must cope with these circumstances or is constantly enervated by them, his or her responses to emotions are indeed likely to be less than optimal. Finally, maltreated children's own patterns of expressiveness are more negative; they exhibit more anger, sadness, and fear than nonmaltreated children. These problematic patterns, if they persist, do not bode well for these children's later social competence (see Chapter 6). More research is needed on this last area, but it would seem evident that maltreated youngsters should benefit from interventions focused on the development of emotional competence.

## Parental Affective Disturbance and Emotional Competence

Parental affective disturbance is another conceivable disrupter of the typical course of emotional development. In particular, maternal depression has been much studied in recent years. Although much anger is expressed, just as in maltreating families, the main characteristics of these affective environments are the sadness, hopelessness, and inappropriate role reversal to which young children are exposed. Mothers' examination of photographs of emotionally expressive infants with their children, and simulations of their own sadness, highlight important aspects of this affective environment (Zahn-Waxler et al., 1993). Depressed mothers focus on their own sorrow, pointing to their children as the cause; in fact, some mothers get so caught up in the simulation that they are unable to bring the episode to resolution. Immersion in such distress on a chronic basis can obviously affect growing preschoolers' developing emotional competence.

In terms of patterns of emotional expressiveness, these children's atypical overinvolvement in interpersonal distress and conflict is conducive to the development of many enduring negative emotions, including potentially incapacitating guilt (Zahn-Waxler & Kochanska, 1990). Toddlers are already absorbing their depressed mothers' explicit and implicit coaching about emotions, contingent reactions to their emotions, and modeling of the negative affect in which the mothers are immersed. Imagine the double bind of this experience: "I am sad, just like Mommy. But if I show my sadness, I upset her. I have to take care of her, because she said she is so-oo sad. Maybe it is my fault, because I act sad." Later in the preschool period, 5-year-olds of depressed mothers showed more overt behavioral difficulties associated with emotional competence deficits—a preponderance of anger and aggression, as well as inability to interact with peers (Denham, Zahn-Waxler, Cummings, & Iannotti, 1991; Zahn-Waxler et al., 1988).

Findings also indicate that young children who live in an environment of depression have difficulties in regulating their own emotional expressiveness. These obstacles can take several forms. Two-year-olds of depressed versus nondepressed mothers cope differently in an emotionally charged situation: When confronted with escalating episodes of argument, conflict, and distress between experimenters, the depressed mothers' children are unusually well behaved, but also significantly more preoccupied and upset than the children of nondepressed mothers. Children of depressed mothers seem to suppress negative emotions, but have trouble regulating them once they are expressed. They almost overuse peacekeeping, comforting, and appeasement as coping strategies, act polite in the face of frustration, and demonstrate less aggression than do the children of nondepressed mothers (Cummings, Iannotti, & Zahn-Waxler, 1985; Denham, Zahn-Waxler, et al., 1991; Zahn-Waxler, McKnew, Cummings, Davenport, & Radke-Yarrow, 1984).

In summary, living in an affectively disordered family environment is very likely to engender both quantitative and qualitative disturbances in preschoolers' developing emotional competence (see, e.g., Thompson, 1994; Thompson & Calkins, 1996). Nonetheless, the accumulating body of evidence has many gaps, especially in these children's understanding of emotions and in clear descriptions of their ER. Furthermore, all three of the emotion socialization pathways—modeling, contingency, and coaching—need to be explicitly and thoroughly investigated for preschoolers with affectively disturbed parents.

## MIXED CONTRIBUTIONS

### "Risk" Status

At times it is not clear whether biological contributions, environmental contributions, or both have provoked observed deficits in emotional competence. Even when clearly defined factors such as autism, developmental disability, maltreatment, or parental affective disturbance are not present, children can be clearly "at risk" for delays in emotional competence. Myriad converging circumstances can contribute to this risk, such as those likely to exist in environments that are traditionally considered "disadvantaged."

Qualitative analyses of year-long observations suggest that "at-risk" preschoolers often express emotions impulsively as felt (Burton & Denham, in press). Particularly troublesome is the inability to understand emotions consciously, in order to solve problems that occur with peers (Burton & Denham, in press; see also Cicchetti, Toth, & Bush, 1988). Such children also have few means of regulating emotions, in part because they have no experience in attaching labels to internal feelings and therefore do not bring their own or others' feelings to consciousness (Greenberg, DeKlyen, & Speltz, 1989).

Understanding and regulating affect are so vital to social relationships that such children are at a distinct disadvantage. If the children do not recognize feelings in themselves, they certainly cannot empathize with the feelings seen in others. They may take a toy out of the hands of another without consideration for the other person, or push another child away simply because that child is in the way of a desired goal. When provoked by another child, these children generally respond with unregulated anger and physical aggression. Angry and without coping strategies, they hit back without thinking, and cannot glean the social advantages of emotional competence.

Hence, "at-risk" status during the preschool period is associated with numerous potential deficits in the development of emotional competence. Clearly, however, more work needs to be done to determine the specific composition of these vulnerabilities. Part of the problem here is that investigators sometimes use rather sloppy definitions of "risk" status; clearer operationalizations are necessary.

## Disruptive Behavior Disorders

More clearly diagnosed behavior disorders constitute a definite threat to the development of emotional competence. The environment of behaviorally disordered children is often emotionally atypical, with more negative emotion witnessed and experienced in both family and peer environments (Patterson, Reid, & Dishion, 1992). Hence, it is reasonable to expect that these children's emotional expressiveness, reactions to others' emotions, and coping with their own emotions will be aberrant. In fact, the diagnostic criteria for and characteristics of oppositional defiant disorder and conduct disorder include lack of concern for the feelings of others; lack of guilt or remorse; readily blaming others; irritability and temper outbursts; low frustration tolerance; and, frequently, comorbid anxiety and depression (see Cole, Michel, & Teti, 1994). Various aspects of comorbid anxiety also suggest lack of emotional competence—unrealistic persistence of worry and fear, as well as marked timidity and tension.

Second, the characteristics of these children suggest compromised emotion understanding. Behaviorally disordered children spend less time scanning their social environment and hence do not pick up on affective information emanating from other people. They also have social-cognitive biases that prevent them from processing emotional cues accurately (see Dodge & Frame, 1982). More and more research suggests that older children with behavioral difficulties tend to see others' behavior with a hostile attribution bias, for example; this can lead to misplaced anger that begins a chain of disturbed interactions. They think that other people mean them harm, and as the prototype and functional analyses of emotion suggest, such a lens for viewing the world leads to their own anger and hampers their social interactions. Even nondiagnosed preschoolers with such biases fare more poorly in their peer setting (Barth & Bastiani, 1997).

More detailed investigations of earlier emotional competence precursors of behavior disorders are now underway (Cole & Zahn-Waxler, 1988; Cole, Zahn-Waxler, & Smith, 1994). In Cole and colleagues' work, preschool-age children at risk for conduct disorder, as well as those not at risk, were observed while a disappointing gift was given to them. Boys who were at risk for conduct disorder showed more negative emotion in the experimenter's presence than low-risk boys did. Their negative emotions (particularly anger) were associated with their overall disruptiveness during the paradigm, as well as with their overall symptomatology.

In contrast, the high-risk preschool girls differed from the low-risk girls after the experimenter left; they actually displayed *less* negative emotion at this point. Their minimization of negative emotion predicted symptoms of attention-deficit/hyperactivity disorder (ADHD) and conduct disorder—overactivity, difficulty concentrating, immaturity, lying, and destructiveness. The authors hypothesize that these girls overregulated their expression of negative emotion, because of the undesirability of negative affect in girls. This overregulation absorbed their attentional resources and behavioral control.

In essence, then, young boys at risk for conduct disorder differed from their low-risk peers in the anger they showed in the presence of the person who caused it. In contrast, young girls at risk for conduct disorder differed from their low-risk counterparts in their overregulation. Both showed exaggerated, nonadaptive patterns of gender-stereotyped emotional expressiveness. Similarly, children in this investigation who were either inexpressive or highly expressive during a negative mood induction showed more externalizing symptoms (Cole, Zahn-Waxler, Fox, Usher, & Welsh, 1996).

Examining longitudinal diagnostic data from the same project, my colleagues and I (Denham, Cole, Weissbrod, Workman, & Zahn-Waxler, 1998) have found that mothers' ratings of preschoolers' temperamental qualities of emotional intensity and negativity predicted externalizing and internalizing problems 1 year later. Overall, then, expressiveness patterns and ability to regulate emotions differ for preschoolers who already exhibit behavior problems commensurate with an ultimate diagnosis of conduct disorder.

Similarly, grade-school-age children with diagnoses of oppositional defiant disorder and/or ADHD showed deficits in emotional competence (Casey & Schlosser, 1994). They were observed interacting with a partner in a game-playing setting, and were interviewed about their emotion understanding; their parents completed questionnaires regarding their children's sensitivity to social feedback. Each diagnostic group showed specific deviations from the expressiveness patterns of nondiagnosed children. The oppositional defiant children showed a limited range of facial expression, primarily negative; their verbalizations and vocal tones were also more hostile while they played the game, compared to those of nondiagnosed children. Children with ADHD showed more facial affect and more frequent changes in facial expression, and used more positive expressiveness during social approach. Furthermore, when ADHD and aggressiveness coexist, boys are characteristically very emotionally negative, and this negativity contributes to peer rejection (Henshaw & Melnick, 1995). Importantly, Casey and Schlosser found that children who managed to exhibit age-appropriate emotional competence skills also scored higher on social competence measures.

Some pertinent findings also exist on older behavior-disordered children's understanding of emotions. First- and second-graders who were rated as higher in behavior problems by parents and teachers showed deficits in emotional understanding on the Kusché Affective Interview (Cook, Greenberg, & Kusché, 1994). On this interview, children are asked to cite personal examples of 10 different emotions, as well as the information used for recognition of five emotions in themselves and others. Children exhibiting teacher- or parent-rated behavior problems showed deficits in both aspects of emotion understanding.

However, intellectual functioning, which was negatively associated with behavior problems, also attenuated the effects of such problems on emotion understanding. In this case, intellectual competence buffered deficits in emotional competence; compensating factors in one domain of development can mitigate deficits in another. Children who can think flexibly are better able to consider emotional issues, despite the disruptive effects of their own behavior. Although it is exciting to find such a resilience factor, its discovery by no means weakens the problems most children with behavior disorders exhibit in the area of emotion understanding.

Deficits in emotion understanding were also exhibited by the behavior-disordered children in Casey and Schlosser's (1994) work. Both diagnosis groups frequently misreported their own recent expressive behavior. Moreover, oppositional defiant children made overly negative interpretations of others' feelings. Children with ADHD made the opposite sort of error—overly positive interpretations of others' feelings. These children misunderstood their own and others' emotions.

Finally, Arsenio and Fleiss (1996) have shown that older behavior-disordered children exhibit a developmentally young social-cognitive bias about moral emotion. They assume the "happy victimizer" position, asserting that a person who has made a peer feel bad may still feel good rather than sorry, because the person has achieved his or her own goal. This pattern of understandings is appropriate to younger children (Lemerise et al., 1996).

As is true of developmentally disabled children, ER has really not been studied in behavior-disordered children. However, given researchers' emphasis on ER for this group (e.g., Cole, Michel, & Teti, 1994), and the crystallization of research in emotional competence as a whole, I am optimistic that useful information will soon be unearthed regarding behavior-disordered children and ER.

Disruptions within the child, the environment, or both are often associated with patterns of deficits in emotional competence. Nonetheless, many gaps in our knowledge of both the emotional strengths and weaknesses of children who experience these disruptions remain to be filled. Given the importance of emotional competence to success in the peer world, it is especially important for the parents, teachers, and caregivers of children with varying problems to do what they can to identify children with special needs in the area of emotional competence, and to foster its growth. To this end, I next describe ways to assess strengths and weaknesses in emotional competence within the preschool period. I then discuss existing intervention programs that directly address milestones of emotional competence.

## MEANS OF ASSESSING YOUNG CHILDREN'S
## EMOTIONAL COMPETENCE

Developmental assessment—whether for screening, diagnosis, or program planning—obviously must be an evaluation of the whole child, not just his or her emotional competence. But assessment of emotional competence is vital and too often overlooked. We are obligated to identify the delays in emotional competence caused by the contributors reviewed above, because these deficits so severely compromise a young child's functioning in the social world. Unfortunately, tools for directly assessing emotional competence are somewhat sparse. Our recent review (Denham, Lydick, Mitchell-Copeland, & Sawyer, 1996) enumerates possible tools for screening, diagnosis, and program planning for children in the toddler and preschool age ranges. The following summary also describes these tools.

Screening tools specifically addressing emotional competence, sometimes along with social competence, include the Denver Developmental Screening Test (DDST; Frankenburg, Camp, & Van Natta, 1971; Frankenburg, Dodds, Fandal, Kazuk, & Cohrs, 1975), the Tool Use Task (Matas, Arend, & Sroufe, 1978; Crowell & Feldman, 1988), and the Minnesota Preschool Affect Checklist (MPAC; Sroufe et al., 1984). Assessment instruments more specifically useful in the diagnosis of emotional competence deficits include the Functional Emotional Assessment Scale for Infancy and Early Childhood (FEASIE; Greenspan, 1992, 1994; this instrument is also useful for program planning) and the two forms of the Child Behavior Checklist (CBCL/2–3 and CBCL/4–16; Achenbach, Edelbrock, & Howell, 1987; Achenbach, 1991). I now discuss the use of these and a few other instruments for the toddler and preschool age ranges. It should be noted that despite our efforts to discover assessment tools that answer questions about the major social-emotional tasks of each age period, the tools available do not always clearly or solely address emotional expressiveness, understanding, and regulation.

## Screening

### Denver Developmental Screening Test

Only two social-emotional items appear on the DDST for the toddler and preschool age ranges: playing interactive games and separating easily from the mother. According to DDST scoring conventions, however, failure of these two items at the toddler age range should not be considered as problematic for this domain of development unless earlier milestones have also been failed. Nonetheless, it is encouraging to note that two major social-emotional tasks of the period are in fact covered by the DDST. Of course, neither of these tasks maps specifically onto emotional competence as I conceptualize it here.

## Research-Based Measures

Research tasks can also be used in an ecologically valid manner to capture many of the important aspects of social-emotional development during this period. Matas et al. (1978) and Crowell and Feldman (1988) have developed the Tool Use Task for children in the 18- to 54-month age group. Faced with four difficult problems after free-play and cleanup periods, plus a separation and reunion in the preschool version, the competent child is seen as enthusiastic and persistent. Symbolic play, oppositionality, compliance, active noncompliance and ignoring, verbal negativism, frustration behavior, aggression, whining/crying, help seeking, enthusiasm, positive/negative affect, and non-task-related behavior are rated. Several of these indices reflect emotional expressiveness and reactions to others' emotions. Concurrent and predictive validity, and interrater and internal-consistency reliability for some of these scales, are described in Denham, Renwick, and Holt (1991) as well as in Matas et al. (1978). The procedures are not difficult to stage or to score.

## Minnesota Preschool Affect Checklist

When more time is available to observe a child within the peer social milieu, the MPAC (Sroufe et al., 1984) is useful to summarize aspects of emotional competence. The developmental tasks on the MPAC include the expression and regulation of positive and negative affect, productive involvement in purposeful activity, impulse control and management of frustration, interaction with peers, and ability to respond prosocially to the emotions of others. For each observation period, observers note the presence or absence of items included within these overarching developmental tasks. The items do a good job of sampling the skills for this age period. The MPAC has demonstrated reliability and validity for this age level (see also Denham, Zahn-Waxler, et al., 1991). It definitely captures elements of expressiveness and coping with one's own and others' emotions, but only one item indirectly addresses understanding of emotions.

## Summary

Across these three screening measures, coverage of the three important elements of emotional competence, as defined here, is spotty and somewhat indirect. I would argue for adapting the Tool Use Task as a middle ground between the quick but relatively uninformative DDST and the rich but time-consuming MPAC. Clearly, there is still a need for a complex, detailed instrument that nevertheless fulfills a screening function. After screening identifies a problem in emotional competence, more detailed diagnostic information is required.

## Diagnosis

### Forms of the Child Behavior Checklist

The CBCL/2–3 (see also the CBCL/4–16) was designed to extend previously developed empirically based assessment procedures (Achenbach, 1991; Achenbach et al., 1987). The measure is completed by parents. Its six empirically derived syndromes are Social Withdrawal, Depressed, Sleep Problems, Somatic Problems, Aggressive, and Destructive; there are also broad-band Internalizing and Externalizing groupings. The psychometric properties of the CBCL/2–3 are excellent, in the tradition of empirically based measures. But this measure, like others of its ilk, is much better for gross screening of pathology than for pinpointing emotional competence. Second, the measure is less comprehensive than the CBCL/4–16. Hence, given these strengths and weaknesses, it might be recommended for initial gross diagnosis and for initial phases of treatment plans. In terms of emotional competence, the two forms if the CBCL really only address expressiveness and, tangentially, reactions to others' emotions.

### Preschool Socioaffective Profile

For diagnostic coverage of both positive and negative social-emotional milestones during the preschool period, the Preschool Socioaffective Profile (PSP) is more useful (LaFreniere & Dumas, 1996; LaFreniere, Dumas, Capuano, & Dubeau, 1992). It targets behaviors reflecting emotional expression in social interaction with peers and adults, along with characteristic emotions in nonsocial context, and thus is a good measure of emotional expressiveness and ER. Of its 30 items, 7 capture emotional expressiveness and 7 illustrate ER, whereas only 1 exemplifies emotion understanding.

Psychometrically speaking, the PSP has excellent interrater, internal-consistency, and test–retest reliability. Three factors have been isolated from the PSP's items: Social Competence, Externalizing behavior, and Internalizing behavior. Concurrent validation of these factors both broad and narrow-band measures of the CBCL/4–16, as well as with observations of social behavior and peer sociometrics, is excellent. Because this measure provides a picture of specific types of problems as well as positive social adaptation, it assists teachers and parents in understanding a child's strengths and weaknesses. Moreover, it is sensitive to behavioral change over time and thus can be used to evaluate intervention outcomes.

## Summary

The PSP can contribute fairly directly to decision making about what to do for a child with complex strengths and weaknesses in emotional competence. It is unfortunate, however, that only one assessment tool for this age range really taps emotional competence. After diagnosis by whatever means, very comprehensive objectives are needed for program planning; further, even ongoing, assessment is called for.

## Program Planning

### Hawaii Early Learning Profile

The Hawaii Early Learning Profile (HELP; Parks, 1992) is designed to be used in program planning for young children who are delayed, have disabilities, or are considered "at risk." HELP items assess preselected play and daily living activities. Professionals report qualitative descriptions of behaviors within all major domains of development, including Social-Emotional; approximate developmental age levels for each behavior are given. The descriptions of children's behaviors and abilities derived from the HELP aid families, early childhood educators, and clinicians in curriculum planning; enable identification of strengths and weaknesses; and facilitate monitoring of children's progress in small incremental steps. HELP's Social-Emotional strand consists of the following subscales: Attachment/Separation/Autonomy, Development of Self, Expression of Emotions and Feelings, Learning Rules and Expectations, and Social Interactions and Play. Each of these subscales includes items appropriate from birth to age 3. Some of the items for each subscale with the 18- to 36-month age range are as follows (Parks, 1992, pp. 280–321):

ATTACHMENT/SEPARATION/AUTONOMY

Displays dependent behavior; clings/whines
Feels strongly possessive of loved ones
Separates easily in familiar surroundings
Shows independence
Insists on doing things independently

### DEVELOPMENT OF SELF

Uses own name to refer to self
Experiences a strong sense of self-importance
Recognizes self in photographs
Uses "self-centered" pronouns
Values own property
Distinguishes self as a separate person; contrasts self with others
Takes pride in achievements

### EXPRESSION OF EMOTIONS AND FEELINGS

Expresses affection
Shows jealousy at attention given to others, especially other family
    members
Shows a wide variety of emotions (e.g., fear, anger, sympathy,
    modesty, guilt, joy)
Feels easily frustrated
Attempts to comfort others in distress
Tantrums peak
Dramatizes feelings using a doll
Fatigues easily
May develop sudden fears, especially of large animals
Demonstrates extreme emotional shifts and paradoxical responses

### LEARNING RULES AND EXPECTATIONS

Desires control of others—orders, fights, resists
Demonstrates awareness of class routines
Says "no," but submits anyway
Dawdles and procrastinates
Begins to obey and respect simple rules
Resists change; is extremely ritualistic
Experiences difficulty with transitions

### SOCIAL INTERACTIONS AND PLAY

Interacts with peers using gestures
Engages in parallel play
Defends possessions
Displays shyness with strangers and in outside situations
Tends to be physically aggressive
Enjoys a wide range of relationships
Relates best to one familiar adult at a time
Engages best in peer interaction with just one older child, not a
    sibling

Initiates own play, but requires supervision to carry out ideas
Tends to be dictatorial and demanding
Participates in . . . interactive games

Clearly not all of these items correspond to expressiveness, understanding of emotions, and ER, but many do. The HELP items are well
organized and sufficiently detailed to be useful in planning for preschoolers with deficits in emotional competence. One possible difficulty
that I see is determining when "too much" of any type of expressive
or regulatory strategy exists (e.g., shyness), despite its developmental
appropriateness.

### Functional Emotional Assessment Scale for Infancy and Early Childhood

A second measure, Greenspan's (1992) FEASIE, represents a more
clinical viewpoint, because it "emphasizes understanding the infant and
young child's emotional and social functioning in the context of
relationships with his or her caregivers and family" (p. 381), and is tied
to Greenspan's theory of emotional development. It can be useful for
both diagnosis and program planning. It is actually a component of a
larger, developmentally based diagnostic classification system of mental
health and developmental disorders of infancy and early childhood
(Emde, Bingham, & Harmon, 1993; Greenspan, 1994; National Center
for Clinical Infant Programs, 1993).

Free, unstructured interaction between the infant or child and his
or her caregiver, as well as the clinician, is the setting for FEASIE
assessment. Quantitative, but not standardized, scores at each level are
used as summaries for the Primary Emotional Capacities and Emotional Range (Sensorimotor and Affective). Because of the issue of
nonstandardization, and also because of the small illustrative sample
potentially biased toward the majority culture, Greenspan asserts that
these scores should be used only for descriptive purposes. Nonetheless,
the categories used in the scale can be rated reliably and do discrimi-
nate between clinical and nonclinical groups. The goal of the FEASIE
is to "assist the clinician in systematizing and fine-tuning clinical
judgments" (Greenspan, 1992, p. 388); it yields a profile that alerts early
childhood clinicians and educators to explore an infant's strengths and
weaknesses in greater depth, thus creating direct links to intervention.
So far, however, although the complex clinical judgments to which
Greenspan refers are operationalized, the FEASIE does not go so far
as to tie them to specific intervention objectives. This work remains to
be done.

So, as it stands now, the FEASIE is a promising planning tool. It
specifies the following objectives for the toddler and preschool age

ranges; much of their intent is to address issues of emotional expression, understanding of emotions, and ER.

1. By 18 months, the infant can elaborate complex, lengthy sequences of interaction that convey basic emotional themes, including aggression and limit setting (Greenspan, 1992, pp. 400–402). Greenspan (1994, p. 39) calls this ability "representational/affective communication."

2. By 24 months, the child can create mental representations of feelings and ideas that can be expressed symbolically (e.g., pretend play and words to convey emotional themes), and he or she can use these to communicate about basic intentions, wishes, needs, or feelings (Greenspan, 1992, pp. 403–404).

3. By 30 months, the child can use symbolic communication and make-believe play to elaborate a number of ideas that go beyond basic needs and deal with more complex intentions, wishes, or feelings (e.g., expressing pride; Greenspan, 1992, p. 406). Greenspan (1994, p. 39) calls this ability "representational elaboration."

4. By 36 months, ideas dealing with complex intentions, wishing, and feelings in pretend play or other types of symbolic communication are now logically tied to one another. The child can distinguish what is real from the unreal, and switches back and forth between fantasy and reality with little difficulty (Greenspan, 1992, p. 408). Greenspan (1994) calls this the first level of "representational differentiation."

5. After 42 months, the child is capable of even more elaborate complex pretend play and symbolic communication dealing with complex intentions, wishes, or feelings. The play or direct communication is characterized by three or more ideas that are logically connected and informed by concepts involving causality, time, and space (Greenspan, 1992, p. 411). Emotional themes now include separation and loss. This is the second, more mature level of representational differentiation.

So, as a diagnostic and program planning tool, the FEASIE plumbs some elements of emotional competence. Continued refinement may yield a useful assessment tool.

## Summary

Program planning measures such as the HELP or the FEASIE need to lead more directly to intervention, and their criterion-referenced, nonstandardized nature may also need to be modified. A more extensive, standardized measure may be called for. Furthermore, the lack of specific intervention objectives that address developmentally appropriate tasks for emotional competence needs to be addressed. In short, better assessment tools that comprehensively pinpoint emotional competence skills—or, at the very least, refinements of those that do exist—are crucially needed.

## INTERVENTIONS TO AMELIORATE DEFICITS IN YOUNG CHILDREN'S EMOTIONAL COMPETENCE

When some aspect of the development of emotional expressiveness, understanding of emotion, or ER is hindered during the preschool years—whether because of contributions from the child or the environment, or some mixture of the two—interventions are necessary. If potential problems have been flagged because of these conditions, and appropriate assessment of emotional competence has been conducted (to the extent that this is possible), then intervention should naturally emerge.

In a special needs preschool setting that serves children with developmental delays and disabilities, there may be a child with autistic tendencies who has particular difficulty attending to emotional cues in his environment. Another child, with a history of physical abuse, may be a member of the class because of identified cognitive and language delays; however, her episodes of freezing when her peers express anger, alternating with her own unbridled expressions of rage, also concern her teacher. A third child in the class may be at risk for significant developmental delay because the conditions of his upbringing—a disadvantaged environment meeting federal, state, and local definitions for subsidized and court-ordered child care—have resulted in real ER difficulties.

Fine-grained interventions, and even primary prevention, targeted at milestones of emotional competence are clearly called for in these cases. Unfortunately, however, most interventionists creating curricula for young children have for years focused on the areas of cognition and language. In fact, few explicit social-emotional curricula exist for any age level. A few attempts, however, have been made. Some of the programs that I now outline address more than one component of emotional competence—expressiveness, understanding of emotion, and/or ER (coping with the emotions of self and others)—but systematic, comprehensive efforts to create curricula for emotional competence are rare.

### Targeting Emotion Understanding Only

Feshbach and Cohen (1988) developed a training program based on the supposition that children's developing understanding of affect in others and in themselves can be facilitated by a systematic educational program. The goals of their curriculum, which recognized the inter-twined roles of affect and cognition in the development of empathy, were to increase children's skill in identifying emotions and their responsiveness to and utilization of emotional cues in others. Although there were only four lessons, they included games that focused on emotional cues, used role playing of a range of emotions, and encour-aged the children to determine how another person would feel in varying situations. Through cognitive self-rehearsal of others' feelings, role play, and songs, the children learned about happiness, sadness, and anger. Children were then tested on emotion identification and description of pictured emotional situations.

Training had little direct effect on emotion identification, but trained children displayed increased sensitivity to and awareness of the feelings of others; they were more able than untrained children to engage in emotional perspective taking. Thus, the intervention was partially successful; perhaps a longer-duration, more extensive interven-tion would have been more useful. Furthermore, a more comprehen-sive intervention that addressed all three areas of emotional competence would have been preferable. In any case, this intervention addressed understanding of emotions, and it could be a springboard for other, more extensive instruction.

## Targeting Emotion Understanding and ER in the Primary Grades

This need for a larger number of more comprehensive, long-lasting lessons has been addressed by at least one group of developmental psychologists. Greenberg, Kusché, Cook, and Quamma (1995; see also Kusché & Greenberg, 1995a) developed a longer-term emotional com-petence curriculum for first- and second-graders. Although it addressed only two of the components of emotional competence,[3] it has potential application for younger children. The stated goals of the intervention were to improve self-control [i.e., ER], emotional understanding, and social problem-solving skills. Much of the curriculum thus focused on thinking about emotions and regulating them. Specific curricular ele-ments included the following:

1. "Stopping and Calming Down," whch focused on controlling emotional arousal and behavior through self-regulation.
2. Enriched linguistic experiences, which were concentrated on mediating the understanding of emotions in self and others.
3. Integrating emotional understanding with cognitive and linguis-

tic skills to analyze and solve problems; children were taught that feelings are signals that communicate useful social information.

4. Developing positive self-esteem and effective peer relations (somewhat outside the scope of the present discussion, but nonetheless related).

Positive outcomes after the 7-month intervention were many. Children receiving the intervention had greater verbal access to affect vocabulary for both positive and negative emotions; gave more appropriate examples of basic and advanced emotions; understood that people can and sometimes should hide feelings, and that feelings change even when a person is upset; and realized that changing bad feelings is possible. There were, however, no effects of intervention on comprehension of the simultaneity of different emotions or on elaborated answers about how, when, and why people hide feelings.

The intervention had extensive impact on the children's understanding of emotions, although some more advanced aspects did not evidence change. Furthermore, although Greenberg and colleagues consider the emotional control step more or less a preparation for what follows, anecdotal reports support its efficacy—a point I return to below.

## Targeting Emotion Understanding and ER in the Preschool Years

Building on the interventions created by Greenberg and colleagues, as well as by Shure and Spivack (1982), we recently implemented a social-emotional prevention program for at-risk 4-year-olds in day care (Denham & Burton, 1996; Burton & Denham, in press). We saw many of these children's risk factors expressed in their emotions, and we were very concerned. There were children who showed precursors of conduct disorder—who were angry and behaviorally out of control. In contrast, there were also withdrawn children, who were quiet, sad, spoke hesitantly, and appeared overwhelmed. Both kinds of social-emotional difficulties often persist after the preschool period (Campbell & Ewing, 1990; Egeland, Kalkoske, Gottesman, & Erickson, 1990), so that early amelioration is sorely needed. These pressing emotional competence needs were directly addressed in this intervention.

Teachers were trained to perform curricular activities over a 32-week period. These activities concentrated on (1) relationship building, (2) emotion understanding, (3) ER, and (4) social problem solving. Although two of these curricular elements do not map directly onto emotional competence as defined here, I describe the intervention in totality because its components were designed to work together, rather than in a piecemeal fashion. As stated previously, I see attainment of a secure attachment relationship with a caregiver as a precursor to the aspects of emotional competence. Furthermore, the social problem-solving capabilities fostered by this intervention can also be seen as social competence outcomes. Accordingly, the components of the curriculum fit well with the conception that emotional competence not only is multifaceted and important in its own right, but also contributes to social competence.

Thus, we developed a program of substantial length to provide attention to emotional competence, as well as a solid foundation of trust, with emphases on social problem solving and individualization. To prevent long-term social-emotional harm in young children at risk, an intervention must address each of these areas.

### Relationship Building

More specifically, regarding relationship building, a day care teacher can develop a relationship with a child that is positive, consistent, and supportive of the growth of emotional competence. In other words, a bond of trust can be forged (van IJzendoorn, Sagi, & Lambermon, 1992; Howes & Matheson, 1992). Children actually seek psychological proximity to teachers when their prior attachment history is insecure (Lynch & Cicchetti, 1992). The building of a relationship between child and teacher was thus the first component of the present intervention process, and served as a foundation for more specifically addressing emotional competence skills.

Teachers used the "floor time" technique as a means of building such a warm and intimate relationship with each child (Greenspan, 1992). To enact this technique during play, they first observed the child, opened communication, and continued the communication process by following the child's lead in play. They then helped the child to expand that play one step further through gestures and words. Through the positive affect sharing and distress relief foci of such an attachment relationship, the seeds are sown for the development of emotional competence.

### Emotion Understanding

To recognize and empathize with the feelings of others, it is important that children be able to recognize these feelings in themselves, label them, and associate them with appropriate physical expressions of affect (Kusché & Greenberg, 1995b). Thus, the second component of the intervention focused on increasing emotion understanding. Preschoolers need to learn that feelings have causes that can be identified, and that behaviors chosen can influence those feelings, both in the self and in others. Without understanding of emotion, no distancing occurs between feeling and action. Our fun lessons in understanding emotions provided these at-risk children with the exposure to feeling words, use of these words to label affect in themselves and in others, and recognition that actions can cause emotions.

## Emotion Regulation

Once feelings are recognized and labeled as they are experienced, a child must learn to regulate the expression of those feelings (Kusché & Greenberg, 1995b). Strong negative feelings, particularly anger, must be recognized as such and then cognitively directed into socially acceptable channels. In our intervention, children were taught a method of controlling these negative feelings called the Turtle Technique (Kusché & Greenberg, 1995a, 1995b; Robin, Schneider, & Dolnick, 1976; Schneider & Robin, 1978). That is, they were encouraged to retreat into their "turtle shell" when they felt hurt or angry. This gave them time to reflect on their feelings and decide how they would react to the cause of these feelings when they came out of their shell. The teacher also talked through the emotions being felt and helped each child express and channel these feelings effectively. These lessons and daily emphases on understanding of emotions and ER reflected a downward extension of the essence of the PATHS curriculum (Kusché & Greenberg, 1995a, 1995b).

## Social Problem Solving and Concomitant Empathy

A fourth component of our program was instruction in social problem solving (Shure & Spivack, 1982, Shure, 1990). In general, this approach promotes adjustment by improving an individual's ability to think through and resolve interpersonal conflicts effectively. The learner is guided to develop habits of generating multiple options and evaluating the effects of these choices on others before acting.

More important for specifically facilitating emotional competence, children's thinking about the effects of their actions upon others also requires the children to develop an active empathy for the feelings of others. The development of such empathy has been somewhat lacking in social problem-solving programs up to now. Because cognitive and affective components of empathy can exist separately (Ridley, Vaughn,

& Wittman, 1982), children may learn to recognize and label emotional states in themselves or others when thinking about the consequences of chosen solutions to interpersonal conflicts, but they still may not "feel as others feel." However, this ability to match feeling states is the hypothesized motivator for positive behavior change; thus young children need to be taught to sympathize, and also to think about regulating their own emotions in the service of getting along with others. Joining emotional competence and social problem solving in the current intervention maximized the likelihood of such empathy and ER.

## Teachers' Implementation of the Program

Implementing relationship building and performing lessons on emotion understanding and social problem solving were not the only vital components of the intervention, however. As asserted by Hyson (1994), we agree that "*planned and impromptu* activities encourage children to talk about . . . and play about emotionally important issues" (p. 84; emphasis added). Many, many aspects of emotional competence can be addressed in the early childhood classroom by first creating a secure emotional environment, then helping children to understand emotions all through the day—modeling genuine, appropriate emotional responses; supporting children's regulation of emotions; and recognizing and honoring children's expressive styles (Hyson, 1994).

So in this intervention teachers were also encouraged to model their own feelings and self-control, and to engage in dialogue with children about solving problems. Each teacher was expected to look for moments during the day when dialoguing techniques could be used to help children think about and apply knowledge about feelings and social problem solving gained during the lessons to their actual play situations. The concentration on emotional competence did not end when lessons were over for the day.

## Outcomes of the Intervention

To quantitatively establish the effectiveness of the program, the children's social-emotional status was assessed via observation (MPAC; see above) and teacher questionnaire (PSP; see above) at the beginning and end of the intervention period. They were compared to a group of children who did not experience the intervention. Children who received the intervention, compared to children who did not receive it, showed decreased emotional negativity over the period. They also showed more productive involvement in ongoing activity, were more able to initiate emotionally positive peer activity, and were seen as improving socially by their teachers. In short, they coped better with their emotions.

Interestingly, children who were most in need of the intervention, as evidenced by low pretest scores, benefited most regarding peer skill, productiveness, and overall teacher-rated social competence. This same finding of targeted improvement has been shown in a Canadian intervention designed for kindergarten students who pretested low on social skill and high on internalizing (Gotlieb et al., 1993; see also Ridley & Bullock, 1984).

Quantitative results of the intervention were gratifying, but qualitative data also showed that children were less negative and more positive in their emotional expressiveness, as well as more adept at understanding and regulating their emotions. Stories related by the children and teachers tell volumes. One little boy, who initially had trouble controlling his anger, had a protracted, heated argument in which he and another child negotiated difficulty over ownership of a toy. He proudly announced, "See, I used my words, not my hands!" Another boy was frightened at a doctor's appointment and happened to see his teacher; he asked her to please read him the "Turtle Story" because he needed it "right now!" (to help him gain control of scary feelings). She did read it to him, and it helped! Giving these boys tools of emotional competence assisted them during difficult moments. Moreover, qualitative analyses also show that teachers' efforts to make their whole curriculum emotion-centered were vital contributors to individual growth (Burton & Denham, in press).

But what happens after children move on to the primary grades? After progressing into kindergarten, one girl told her former teacher, whom she sought out during extended day care, "I know you taught me to talk instead of hit, but in kindergarten everyone hits. What do I do? Hit back?" Clearly she had absorbed the basic message of this program and was straining to retain it. This youngster's poignant query points to another need for future research: Are these results long-lasting? Can the intervention generalize to new situations, even when those new situations provide no support for lessons learned? It may be that emotional competence has to be supported in an ongoing fashion throughout the early grades.

Some promising interventions for emotional competence thus exist, even though most developmental interventions still highlight more cognitive areas. The interventions described above pinpoint emotional expressiveness, understanding, and coping, but more work remains to be done to fine-tune specific objectives in this area and the means of meeting them. Tighter, more specific assessment tools, directly tied to intervention, would be very useful.

Goleman (1995) has described emotional literacy as understanding and coping with one's own and others' emotions. Helping all children attain emotional literacy is our goal. Ideally, the ideas described as interventions here can and should be primary prevention for every child (see also Hyson, 1994). It is but a small step, too, from primary prevention to the most minute day-to-day interactions between adults and children.

## ADVICE FOR PARENTS AND EARLY CHILDHOOD EDUCATORS

What is the "takeaway message" here? What other practical points can be gleaned from the information covered in this volume? In order to answer this question, I point out what adults need to be aware of in terms of preschoolers' emotional competence, and what they can do to foster it.

### What Adults Need to Be Aware of: Emotional Competence in General

Adults who play important roles in young children's lives need to know how children differ in terms of emotional competence, in order to be able to live harmoniously with them day by day and to help them develop into healthy, productive people. Specifically, caregivers and parents must recognize that there are important developmental and individual differences in preschoolers' emotional competence. If we are to interact with and nurture young children successfully, we need to be prepared for the differences in the emotional makeup between children at any one age level, as well as between children who differ in age.

Furthermore, caregivers need to recognize that despite preschoolers' formidable abilities in emotional competence, limiting factors do exist. For example, before expecting certain levels of understanding of emotion particular expressive patterns, or specific means of ER, it would be wise to consider each individual child's age, as well as his or her intellectual level. Other specific aspects of emotional competence must also be considered.

### Expressiveness

It is vital to keep up with preschoolers' increased emotional sophistication. The increasing subtlety and complexity of preschoolers' emotionality also need to be acknowledged, so that adults in their lives can support their development. For instance, the mother of a 4-year-old-girl needs to be aware when her daughter shows a mixture of sadness and anger when arguing about getting ready for school; this blend has a different meaning than unalloyed defiance does. Assuming that the child is "fine" at school just because she does not appear overtly afraid is also a mistake. Too often adults "barrel ahead" without considering the growing emotional competence of their charges. So adults' accuracy in receiving their young charges' emotional signals, and the subsequent appropriateness of their own emotional signals, are especially important.

The manifestations and implications of toddlers' and preschoolers' new social and self-conscious emotions deserve careful attention. Parents, caregivers, and educators are motivated to promote the experience of sympathy, because of its association with concern and prosocial behavior. Emphasizing the importance of empathy, and distinguishing between the subcomponents of sympathy and personal distress, are first steps. Then, if we can focus in on important parameters of the development of sympathy (e.g., similarity of experience), we can help facilitate children's healthy and rewarding interpersonal relationships.

The important adults in young children's lives will also want to be able to recognize guilt and shame when the children express them, and to act in a supportive manner. They will want to cheer along when the children experience pride. No doubt they will also want to carefully assess their own role in engendering the experience of these complicated emotions.

With respect to embarrassment, caregivers, parents, and early childhood educators can help young children modify their perception that an audience is making fun of them, because of the potential debilitating effects of this belief. In everyday settings, children may think they are being made fun of when they are not. If a preschool boy freezes in fear and embarrassment when asked to sing a song with his classmates, he can be reassured that no one will laugh at him, so that the discomfort of embarrassment can be avoided.

*Understanding*

Adult caregivers can make use of their preschoolers' emotion understanding. For example, they can tailor their help in ER to those strategies that young children best understand. Consider a 5-year-old boy's feelings of great sadness when his pet dies. It may be a good idea for his father to suggest a visit to the amusement park together—after all, sadness *can* turn into happiness. He can also suggest that his son think about his upcoming fun at day camp. But telling him any variation on the theme of "time heals all wounds" will not be worth-while!

The limits of young children's emotion understanding need to be kept in mind as well. Recall that preschoolers do not really discern either guilt or shame as separate emotions; they just feel "sad" about transgression and failures. Parents, teachers, and caregivers need to know that this apparent lag in emotion understanding is perfectly normal, and not an indication of budding sociopathy. Young children are very unlikely to say "I'm guilty" about a transgression, no matter how important it is.

As important as it is to realize what young children do *not* understand about emotions, it is also necessary to think about what they *may* understand. In situations where they can be expected to experience ambivalent emotions, for example, young children may understand their caregivers' appropriate reference to such feelings even if they themselves do not spontaneously comment on them. Imagine a mother acting as if it were the most natural thing in the world for her 5-year-old daughter to feel happy and sad about the end of the school year. She mentions both those feelings in introducing the topic to the child as they drive home from the last day of kindergarten. The girl joins in this discussion freely, in relief; her mother has "hit the nail on the head," opening up talk about emotions that the child could not begin by herself.

### Emotional Regulation

Adults also need to consider how much support preschoolers in general need in order to accomplish ER. Often children under six need the comfort of a lap to soothe the physiological arousal of sadness or fear, a quiet conversation with a parent to give a name to their disquietude, and a big person's ideas about what to do about an emotional experience. As noted earlier (Chapter 5), preschoolers are taking their first small steps toward handling ER processes on their own.

In addition, particular preschoolers may have more or less ease in either supported or independent ER. Highly reactive children (who are easy to recognize!) need more support in their ER, and may need their supporters to be especially skillful in picking ER strategies tailored to their needs. A little girl whose latency to express fear around animals is extremely short, accompanied by high intensity arousal and long recovery time, may be best served by an adult companion who plans ahead to avoid such situations and has a few tried-and-true means to help her feel better. A boy who is very *un*reactive may need an equally skillful adult to help him discern the mild arousal he does experience as emotion.

In short, ER is an area where adult partners are often vital, across contexts and emotions. It is also important for adults to be attuned to ER and to know their children can manage alone. An intrusive adult could have disrupted the fruitful ER "practice" of a girl who was quite capable of soothing her own ankle. As in any partnership, balance is the key.

## What Adults Can Do: Socialization Practices Specific to Emotional Competence

Let me reiterate the gist of the model put forward in Figure 1.2. Parents and all other adults with whom young children interact—through their own emotions, the ways they react to the children's emotions, and they ways they teach about emotions—affect vital emotional competence that is developing during the preschool years. Furthermore, I think that children who understand emotions better, show more positive emotions, and regulate the "tougher" emotions are seen by preschool teachers as more socially able, are better liked by their peers, and can respond more appropriately to their friends' feelings. So adults are vitally important in this area.

Overall, caregivers' emotions, reactions to kids' emotions, and teaching about emotions wield a potent "double whammy": They affect both emotional and social competence. And what a child practices in terms of emotional competence with adults translates to the realm of peers. So these conclusions reached from the current state of research should give caregivers and parents pause. For preschoolers' benefit, important adults can make adjustments in their own expressiveness and their reactions to children's emotions. Parents and caregivers can also benefit from more careful consideration of, and from open (though not overwhelming) discussions of, their own feelings. Here is more detail on what has been learned so far. For economy, I use the word "parents," but I really mean any important adults with whom children have a relationship.

### PARENTS' EXPRESSIVENESS

• Children whose parents are more emotionally positive tend to be more positive themselves around their peers, whereas children whose parents are more negative appear less socially competent in preschool.

• Parents who report that they can remain emotionally positive during challenging circumstances have children who are more adept at understanding emotions. These findings include dads!

• Young girls' ability to regulate negative emotions is especially vulnerable to the detrimental effects of parents' negative emotions and parents' "mean" reactions to their emotions, as well as to the positive effects of parents' own positive emotions. Little girls are exquisite barometers of parents' emotions. This may be both a blessing and a curse!

### PARENTS' COACHING ABOUT EMOTIONS

• Parents who are better coaches of their children's emotions have children who understand emotions better and are more socially competent in preschool. Talking about feelings is vital. (Not surprisingly, though, some of this depends on whether the child is younger or older during the preschool years, and whether the child is male or female.)

• However, parents' use of guiding and socializing emotion language is a negative predictor of both emotional and social competence. Parents use guiding language (e.g., "You really made me sad that time; I wish you wouldn't scream like that") and socializing language (e.g., "Big kids don't cry so much") with children who most actively need such teaching, such as those who are more prone to exhibit sadness and fear, to react immaturely to others' emotions, or to experience more difficult social relations. Preschoolers may also be "wise" to being bullied or preached at via emotion language, so not all emotion talk is created equal!

### PARENTS' REACTIONS TO CHILDREN'S EMOTIONS

• Parental reactions to children's own emotional displays are important, because children generalize them to their own expressiveness and use them in building emotion knowledge. For example, discouragement of a child's emotion (e.g., by saying "Stop that crying!") is a powerful deterrent of self-reflection regarding emotions, and hence a barrier to emotion knowledge.

• Paying attention to and positively reinforcing children's emotions by accepting them, acknowledging them, and responding to meet the children's pragmatic needs may pave the way for children to learn more about their own and others' emotions, as reflected in their social competence.

The ways we pay attention to, understand, and promote emotional competence in the early years will reap incalculable rewards. It is my fervent hope that we begin now to act upon this knowledge.

# NOTES

1. But see Phillips, Baron-Cohen, and Rutter (1995) for evidence that even understanding of volition (i.e., desire) is impaired in autistic individuals.
2. Avoiding facial cues of emotions makes it difficult, if not impossible, for autistic children to react to the person emitting the emotion. S. T. Auerbach-Major (personal communication, 1997) reports recent success in improving autistic children's understanding of others' emotion when my puppet procedure is used as a training, rather than an assessment, tool.
3. The criticism that ER, but not expressiveness, was captured by this (and the next) intervention may be unfair, in that if ER is facilitated, expressiveness patterns are also no doubt altered.

# References

Abraham, K. G., Kuehl, R. O., & Christopherson, V. A. (1983). Age-specific influence of parental behaviors on the development of empathy in preschool children. *Child Study Journal, 13*, 175–185.

Abramovitch, R., & Daly, E. M. (1979). Inferring attributes of a situation from the facial expressions of peers. *Child Development, 50*, 586–589.

Achenbach, T. M. (1991). *Manual for the Child Behavior Checklist/4–16 and 1991 Profile*. Burlington: University of Vermont, Department of Psychiatry.

Achenbach, T. M., & Edelbrock, C. S. (1986). *Child Behavior Checklist and Youth Self-Report*. Burlington: University of Vermont, Department of Psychiatry.

Achenbach, T. M., Edelbrock, C. S., & Howell, C. T. (1987). Empirically based assessment of the behavioral/emotional problems of 2- and 3-year-old children. *Journal of Abnormal Child Psychology, 15*, 629–650.

Adams, S., Kuebli, J., Boyle, P. A., & Fivush, R. (1995). Gender differences in parent–child conversations about past emotions: A longitudinal investigation. *Sex Roles, 33*, 309–323.

Alessandri, S. M., & Lewis, M. (1993). Parental evaluation and its relation to shame and pride in young children. *Sex Roles, 29*, 335–343.

Alessandri, S. M., & Lewis, M. (1996). Differences in pride and shame in maltreated and normal preschoolers. *Child Development, 67*, 1857–1870.

Altshuler, J. L., & Ruble, D. N. (1989). Developmental changes in children's awareness of strategies for coping with uncontrollable stress. *Child Development, 60*, 1337–1349.

Arsenio, W. F., & Fleiss, K. (1996). Behavior disordered and atypical children's conceptions of sociomoral affect. *British Journal of Developmental Psychology, 14*, 173–186.

Arsenio, W. F., & Kramer, R. (1992). Victimizers and their victims: Children's conceptions of the mixed emotional consequences of moral transgression. *Child Development, 63,* 915–927.

Arsenio, W. F., & Lover, A. (1995). Children's conceptions of sociomoral affect: Happy victimizers, mixed emotions, and other expressions. In M. Killen & D. Hart (Eds.), *Morality in everyday life: Developmental perspectives* (pp. 87–128). New York: Cambridge University Press.

Arsenio, W. F., & Lover, A. (1997). Emotions, conflicts, and aggression during preschoolers' freeplay. *British Journal of Developmental Psychology, 15,* 531–542.

Arsenio, W. F., Lover, A., Cooperman, J., Fein, A., Gordy, A., & Preiser, L. (1997). Emotions, conflicts, and preschoolers' peer acceptance. In J. Hubbard (Chair), *The role of emotions in children's peer relationships.* Symposium conducted at the biennial meeting of the Society for Research in Child Development, Washington, DC.

Auerbach-Major, S. T., Kochanoff, A. T., & Queenan, P. (1997). *The interactive contributions of child temperament and parent disciplinary style on preschoolers' social competence.* Poster presented at the biennial meeting of the Society for Research in Child Development, Washington, DC.

Band, E. B., & Weisz, J. R. (1988). How to feel better when it feels bad: Children's perspectives on coping with everyday stress. *Developmental Psychology, 24,* 247–253.

Banerjee, M. (1997a). Hidden emotions: Preschoolers' knowledge of appearance–reality and emotion display rules. *Social Cognition, 15,* 107–132.

Banerjee, M. (1997b). Peeling the onion: A multi-layered view of children's emotional development. In S. Hala (Ed.), *The development of social cognition* (pp. 241–272). London: Psychology Press.

Banerjee, M., & Eggleston, R. (1993). *Preschoolers' and parents' understanding of emotion regulation.* Poster presented at the biennial meeting of the Society for Research in Child Development, New Orleans, LA.

Barden, R. C., Zelko, F. A., Duncan, S. W., & Masters, J. C. (1980). Children's consensual knowledge about the experiential determinants of emotion. *Journal of Personality and Social Psychology, 39,* 968–976.

Barnett, L. A. (1984). Research note: Young children's resolution of distress through play. *Journal of Child Psychology and Psychiatry, 25,* 477–483.

Barnett, M. A. (1984). Similarity of experience and empathy in preschoolers. *Journal of Genetic Psychology, 145,* 241–250.

Barnett, M. A., Howard, J. A., & Melton, E. M. (1982). Effect of inducing sadness about self or other on behavior in high- and low-empathic children. *Child Development, 53,* 920–923.

Barnett, M. A., King, L. M., Howard, J. A., & Dino, G. A. (1980). Empathy in young children: Relation to parents' empathy, affection, and emphasis on feelings of others. *Developmental Psychology, 16,* 243–244.

Baron-Cohen, S. (1991). Do people with autism understand what causes emotion? *Child Development, 62,* 385–395.

Barrett, K. C. (1996). *The measurement of guilt- and shame-relevant responses during toddlerhood*. Paper presented at the biennial meeting of the International Society for Research in Emotions, Toronto.

Barrett, K. C., & Campos, J. J. (1991) A diacritical function approach to emotions and coping. In E. M. Cummings, A. L. Greene, & K. H. Karraker (Eds.), *Lifespan developmental psychology: Perspectives on stress and coping* (pp. 21–41). Hillsdale, NJ: Erlbaum.

Barrett, K. C., Zahn-Waxler, C., & Cole, P. M. (1993). Avoiders versus amenders—Implications for the investigation of guilt and shame during toddlerhood? *Cognition and Emotion, 7,* 481–505.

Barth, J. M., & Bastiani, A. (1997). A longitudinal study of emotional recognition and preschool children's social behavior. *Merrill–Palmer Quarterly, 43,* 107–128.

Batson, C. D. (1991). *The altruism question: Toward a social psychological answer.* Hillsdale, NJ: Erlbaum.

Beaver, B. R. (1997). The role of emotion in children's selection of strategies for coping with daily stresses. *Merrill–Palmer Quarterly, 43,* 129–146.

Beeghly, M., & Cicchetti, D. (1994). Child maltreatment, attachment, and the self-system: Emergence of an internal state lexicon in toddlers at high social risk. *Development and Psychopathology, 6,* 5–30.

Bennett, M. (1989). Children's self-attributions of embarrassment. *British Journal of Developmental Psychology, 7,* 207–217.

Bennett, M., & Gillingham, K. (1991). The role of self-focused attention in children's attributions of social emotions to the self. *Journal of Genetic Psychology, 152,* 303–309.

Bernzweig, J., Eisenberg, N., & Fabes, R. (1993). Children's coping in self- and other-relevant contexts. *Journal of Experimental Child Psychology, 55,* 208–226.

Bischof-Kohler, D. (1988). On the connection between empathy and the ability to recognize oneself in the mirror. *Schweizerische Zeitschrift für Psychologie, 47,* 147–159.

Blurton-Jones, N. (1967). An ethological study of some aspects of social behaviour of children in nursery school. In D. Morris (Ed.), *Primate ethology.* London: Weidenfeld and Nicolson.

Borke, H. (1971). Interpersonal perception of young children: Egocentrism or empathy? *Developmental Psychology, 5,* 263–269.

Boyum, L. A., & Parke, R. D. (1995). The role of family emotional expressiveness in the development of children's social competence. *Journal of Marriage and the Family, 57,* 593–608.

Bowling, B., & Jones, D. C. (1993). *Family expressiveness and display rule knowledge.* In D. C. Jones (Chair), *Emotions and the family.* Symposium conducted at the biennial meeting of the Society for Research in Child Development, New Orleans, LA.

Bretherton, I., & Beeghly, M. (1982). Talking about internal states: The acquisition of an explicit theory of mind. *Developmental Psychology, 18,* 906–921.

Bretherton, I., Fritz, J., Zahn-Waxler, C., & Ridgeway, D. (1986). Learning to talk about emotions: A functionalist perspective. *Child Development, 57,* 529–548.

Bridges, L. J., & Grolnick, W. S. (1994). The development of emotional self-regulation in infancy and early childhood. In N. Eisenberg (Ed.), *Review of personality and social psychology: Vol. 15. Social development* (pp. 185–211). Thousand Oaks, CA: Sage.

Bridges, L. J., & Grolnick, W. S. (1995). *The development of emotional self-regulatory strategies in infancy and early childhood.* Paper presented at the biennial meeting of the Society for Research in Child Development, Indianapolis, IN.

Brody, L. R., & Harrison, R. H. (1987). Developmental changes in children's abilities to match and label emotionally laden situations. *Motivation and Emotion, 11,* 347–365.

Brown, J. R., Donelan-McCall, N., & Dunn, J. (1996). Why talk about mental states?: The significance of children's conversations with friends, siblings, and mothers. *Child Development, 67,* 836–849.

Brown, J. R., & Dunn, J. (1991). "You can cry, Mum": The social and developmental implications of talk about internal states. *British Journal of Developmental Psychology, 9,* 237–256.

Brown, J. R., & Dunn, J. (1992). Talk with your mother or your sibling?: Developmental changes in early family conversations about feelings. *Child Development, 63,* 336–349.

Brown, J. R., & Dunn, J. (1996). Continuities in emotion understanding from three to six years. *Child Development, 67,* 789–802.

Brown, K., Covell, K., & Abramovitch, R. (1991). Time course and control of emotion: Age differences in understanding and recognition. *Merrill–Palmer Quarterly, 37,* 273–287.

Bullock, M., & Russell, J. (1984). Preschool children's interpretations of facial expressions of emotion. *International Journal of Behavioral Development, 7,* 193–214.

Bullock, M., & Russell, J. (1985). Further evidence on preschoolers' interpretation of facial expressions. *International Journal of Behavioral Development, 8,* 15–38.

Bullock, M., & Russell, J. (1986). Conceptual emotions in developmental psychology. In C. E. Izard & P. Read (Eds.), *Measurement of emotions in children* (Vol. 2, pp. 203–237). New York: Cambridge University Press.

Burton, R., & Denham, S. A. (in press). "Are you my friend?": A qualitative analysis of a social-emotional intervention for at-risk four-year-olds. *Childhood Education.*

Butkovsky, L. L. (1991). *Emotional expressiveness in the family: Connection to children's peer relations.* Poster presented at the biennial meeting of the Society for Research in Child Development, Seattle, WA.

Campbell, S., & Ewing, L. J. (1990). Follow-up of hard-to-manage preschoolers: Adjustment at age 9 and predictors of continuing symptoms. *Journal of Child Psychology and Psychiatry, 31,* 871–889.

Campos, J. J., & Barrett, K. C. (1984). Toward a new understanding of emotions and their development. In C. E. Izard, J. Kagan, & R. B. Zajonc (Eds.), *Emotions, cognition, and behavior* (pp. 229–263). Cambridge, England: Cambridge University Press.

Campos, J. J., Campos, R. G., & Barrett, K. C. (1989). Emergent themes in the study of emotional development and emotion regulation. *Developmental Psychology, 25,* 394–402.

Campos, J. J., Mumme, D. L., Kermoian, R., & Campos, R. G. (1994). A functionalist perspective on the nature of emotion. In N. A. Fox (Ed.), The development of emotion regulation: Biological and behavioral considerations. *Monographs of the Society for Research in Child Development, 59*(2–3, Serial No. 240), 284–303.

Camras, L. A., & Allison, K. (1985). Children's understanding of emotional facial expressions and verbal labels. *Journal of Nonverbal Behavior, 9,* 84–94.

Camras, L., Ribordy, S., & Hill, J. (1988). Recognition and posing of emotional expressions by abused children and their mothers. *Developmental Psychology, 24,* 776–781.

Camras, L., Ribordy, S., Hill, J., Martino, S., Sachs, V., Spaccarelli, S., & Stefani, R. (1990). Maternal facial behavior and the recognition and production of emotional expression by maltreated and nonmaltreated children. *Developmental Psychology, 26,* 304–312.

Carlson, C. R., Felleman, E. S., & Masters, J. C. (1983). Influence of children's emotional states on the recognition of emotion in peers and social motives to change another's emotional state. *Motivation and Emotion, 7,* 61–79.

Carson, J., & Parke, R. D. (1996). Reciprocal negative affect in parent–child interactions and children's peer competency. *Child Development, 67,* 2217–2226.

Casey, R. J., & Fuller, L. (1994). Maternal regulation of children's emotions. *Journal of Nonverbal Behavior, 18,* 57–89.

Casey, R. J., Fuller, L., & Johll, T. (1993). *Parental regulation of children's emotional responses: Will wishing make it so?* In D. C. Jones (Chair), *Emotions and the family.* Symposium conducted at the biennial meeting of the Society for Research in Child Development, New Orleans, LA.

Casey, R. J., & Schlosser, S. (1994). Emotional responses to peer praise in children with and without a diagnosed externalizing disorder. *Merrill–Palmer Quarterly, 40,* 60–81.

Cassidy, J., Parke, R. D., Butkovsky, L., & Braungart, J. M. (1992). Family–peer connections: The roles of emotional expressiveness within the family and children's understanding of emotions. *Child Development, 63,* 603–618.

Chapman, M., Zahn-Waxler, C., Cooperman, G., & Iannotti, R. (1987). Empathy and responsibility in the motivation of children's helping. *Developmental Psychology, 23,* 140–145.

Chen, D., Sullivan, M., & Lewis, M. (1995). *Shame and pride, sadness and joy expressions in 4- and 5-year-old children.* Poster presented at the biennial meeting of the Society for Research in Child Development, Indianapolis, IN.

Cheyne, J. A. (1976). Development of forms and functions of smiling in preschoolers. *Child Development, 47,* 820–823.

Cicchetti, D., Toth, S., & Bush, M. (1988). Developmental psychopathology and incompetence in childhood: Suggestions for intervention. In B. Lahey & A. Kazdin (Eds.), *Advances in clinical child psychology* (pp. 1–72). New York: Plenum Press.

Cole, P. M. (1985). Display rules and the socialization of affective displays. In G. Zivin (Ed.), *The development of expressive behavior* (pp. 269–290). New York: Academic Press.

Cole, P. M. (1986). Children's spontaneous control of facial expressions. *Child Development 57*, 1309–1321.

Cole, P. M., Barrett, K. C., & Zahn-Waxler, C. (1992). Emotion displays in two-year-olds during mishaps. *Child Development, 63*, 314–324.

Cole, P. M., Michel, M. K., & Teti, L. O. (1994). The development of emotion regulation and dysregulation: A clinical perspective. In N. A. Fox (Ed.), The development of emotion regulation: Biological and behavioral considerations. *Monographs of the Society for Research in Child Development, 59*(2–3, Serial No. 240), 73–102.

Cole, P. M., & Zahn-Waxler, C. (1988). *Prediction of conduct problems during the transition from preschool to school age* (Protocol No. 88-M-0217). Bethesda, MD: National Institute of Mental Health.

Cole, P. M., Zahn-Waxler, C., Fox, N. A., Usher, B. A., & Welsh, J. D. (1996). Individual differences in emotion regulation and behavior problems in preschool children. *Journal of Abnormal Psychology, 103*, 518–529.

Cole, P. M., Zahn-Waxler, C., & Smith, K. D. (1994). Expressive control during a disappointment: Variations related to preschoolers' behavior problems. *Developmental Psychology, 30*, 833–846.

Cook, E. T., Greenberg, M. T., & Kusché, C. A. (1994). The relations between emotional understanding, intellectual functioning, and disruptive behavior problems in elementary school aged children. *Journal of Abnormal Child Psychology, 22*, 205–219.

Cortez, V. L., & Bugental, D. B. (1994). Children's visual avoidance of threat: A strategy associated with low social control. *Merrill–Palmer Quarterly, 40*, 82–97.

Costin, S. E., & Jones, D. C. (1992). Friendship as a facilitator of emotional responsiveness and prosocial interventions among young children. *Developmental Psychology, 28*, 941–947.

Covell, K., & Abramovitch, R. (1987). Understanding of emotion in the family: Children's and parents' attributions of happiness, sadness, and anger. *Child Development, 58*, 985–991.

Covell, K., & Abramovitch, R. (1988). Children's understanding of maternal anger: Age and source of anger differences. *Merrill–Palmer Quarterly, 34*, 353–368.

Covell, K., & Miles, B. (1992). Children's beliefs about strategies to reduce parental anger. *Child Development, 63*, 381–390.

Crockenberg, S. B. (1985). Toddlers' reactions to maternal anger. *Merrill–Palmer Quarterly, 31*, 361–373.

Crowell, J. A., & Feldman, S. S. (1988). Mothers' internal working models of relationships' behavioral and developmental status: A study of mother–child interaction. *Child Development, 59*, 1273–1285.

Cummings, E. M. (1987). Coping with background anger in early childhood. *Child Development, 58*, 976–984.

Cummings, E. M. (1995a). Security, emotionality, and parental depression: A commentary. *Developmental Psychology, 31,* 425–427.

Cummings, E. M. (1995b). Usefulness of experiments for the study of the family. *Journal of Family Psychology, 9,* 175–185.

Cummings, E. M., & Cummings, J. L. (1988). A process-oriented approach to children's coping with adult's angry behavior. *Developmental Review, 8,* 296–321.

Cummings, E. M., Hennessy, K. D., Rabideau, G. J., & Cicchetti, D. (1994). Responses of physically abused boys to interadult anger involving their mothers. *Development and Psychopathology, 6,* 31–41.

Cummings, E. M., Iannotti, R. J., & Zahn-Waxler, C. (1985). Influence of conflict between adults on the emotions and aggression of young children. *Developmental Psychology, 21,* 495–507.

Cummings, E. M., Simpson, K. S., & Wilson, A. (1993). Children's responses to interadult anger as a function of information about resolution. *Developmental Psychology, 29,* 978–985.

Cummings, E. M., Zahn-Waxler, C., & Radke-Yarrow, M. (1981). Young children's responses to expressions of anger and affection by others in the family. *Child Development, 52,* 1274–1282.

Cunningham, J. G., & Odom, R. D. (1986). Differential salience of facial features in children's perception of affective expression. *Child Development, 57,* 136–142.

Dadds, M. R., Sanders, M. R., Morrison, M., & Rebetz, M. (1992). Childhood depression and conduct disorder: II. An analysis of family interaction patterns in the home. *Journal of Abnormal Psychology, 101,* 505–513.

Davies, P. T., & Cummings, E. M. (1995). Children's emotions as organizers of their reactions to interadult anger: A functionalist perspective. *Developmental Psychology, 31,* 677–684.

Dawson, G., Hill, D., Spencer, A., Galpert, L., & Watson, L. (1990). Affective exchanges between young autistic children and their mothers. *Journal of Abnormal Child Psychology, 18,* 335–345.

Denham, S. A. (1986). Social cognition, social behavior, and emotion in preschoolers: Contextual validation. *Child Development, 57,* 194–201.

Denham, S. A. (1989). Maternal affect and toddlers' social-emotional competence. *American Journal of Orthopsychiatry, 59,* 368–376.

Denham, S. A. (1993). Maternal emotional responsiveness and toddlers' social-emotional functioning. *Journal of Child Psychology and Psychiatry, 34,* 725–728.

Denham, S. A. (1996a). *Preschoolers' understanding of parents' emotions: Implications for emotional competence.* Unpublished manuscript.

Denham, S. A. (1996b). [Maternal child-rearing practices: Contributions to preschoolers' understanding of emotion.] Unpublished raw data.

Denham, S. A. (1997). "When I have a bad dream, Mommy holds me": Preschoolers' consequential thinking about emotions and social competence. *International Journal of Behavioral Development, 20,* 301–319.

Denham, S. A., & Auerbach, S. (1995). Mother–child dialogue about emotions. *Genetic, Social, and General Psychology Monographs, 121,* 311–338.

Denham, S. A., Auerbach-Major, S., & Blair, K. A. (1997). Preschoolers' emotional competence: Pathway to mental health? In J. Hubbard (Chair), *The role of emotions in children's peer relationships*. Symposium conducted at the biennial meeting of the Society for Research in Child Development, Washington, DC.

Denham, S. A., Blair, K. A., Dixon, R., Schmidt, M. S., & DeMulder, E. (1997). *Compromised emotional competence: Seeds of violence sown early?* Paper presented at the Seventh CHD[3] Annual Conference on Child Development, University of Medicine and Dentistry of New Jersey, New Brunswick.

Denham, S. A., & Burger, C. (1991). Observational validation of teacher rating scales. *Child Study Journal, 21*, 185–202.

Denham, S. A., & Burton, R. (1996). A social-emotional intervention program for at risk four-year-olds. *Journal of School Psychology, 34*, 225–245.

Denham, S. A., Cole, P., Weissbrod, C., Workman, E., & Zahn-Waxler, C. (1998). *Parental and child contributions to externalizing and internalizing patterns in young children at risk for disruptive behavior problems*. Manuscript submitted for revision.

Denham, S. A., Cook, M. C., & Zoller, D. (1992). "Baby looks *very* sad": Discussions about emotions between mother and preschooler. *British Journal of Developmental Psychology, 10*, 301–315.

Denham, S. A., & Couchoud, E. A. (1990a). Young preschoolers' understanding of emotion. *Child Study Journal, 20*, 171–192.

Denham, S. A., & Couchoud, E. A. (1990b). Young preschoolers' understanding of equivocal emotion situations. *Child Study Journal, 20*, 193–202.

Denham, S. A., & Couchoud, E. A. (1991). Social-emotional contributors to preschoolers' responses to an adult's negative emotions. *Journal of Child Psychology and Psychiatry, 32*, 595–608.

Denham, S. A., & Grout, L. (1992). Mothers' emotional expressiveness and coping: Topography and relations with preschoolers' social-emotional competence. *Genetic, Social, and General Psychology Monographs, 118*, 75–101.

Denham, S. A., & Grout, L. (1993). Socialization of emotion: Pathway to preschoolers' affect regulation. *Journal of Nonverbal Behavior, 17*, 205–227.

Denham, S. A., & Holt, R. (1993). Preschoolers' peer status: A cause or consequence of behavior? *Developmental Psychology, 29*, 271–275.

Denham, S. A., Lehman, E. B., Moser, M. H., & Reeves, S. (1995). Continuity and change in emotional components of temperament. *Child Study Journal, 25*, 289–304.

Denham, S. A., Lydick, S., Mitchell-Copeland, J., & Sawyer, K. (1996). Social-emotional assessment for atypical infants and preschoolers. In M. Lewis & M. E. Sullivan (Eds.), *Emotional development in atypical children* (pp. 227–271). Hillsdale, NJ: Erlbaum.

Denham, S. A., & McKinley, M. (1993). Sociometric nominations of preschoolers: A psychometric analysis. *Early Education and Development, 4*, 109–122.

Denham, S. A., McKinley, M., Couchoud, E. A., & Holt, R. (1990). Emotional and behavioral predictors of peer status in young preschoolers. *Child Development, 61*, 1145–1152.

Denham, S. A., Mitchell-Copeland, J., Strandberg, K., Auerbach, S., & Blair, K.

(1997). Parental contributions to preschoolers' emotional competence: Direct and indirect effects. *Motivation and Emotion, 27,* 65–86.

Denham, S. A., Mitchell-Copeland, J., Strandberg, K., & Highsmith, T. (1994, June). Parental contributions to preschoolers' emotional competence: Direct and indirect effects. In G. Pettit & A. Russell (Chairs), *Dimensions and consequences of positive parenting.* Symposium conducted at the biennial meeting of the International Society for the Study of Behavioural Development, Amsterdam.

Denham, S. A., Renwick, S., & Holt, R. (1991). Working and playing together: Prediction of preschool social-emotional competence from mother–child interaction. *Child Development, 62,* 242–249.

Denham, S. A., Renwick-DeBardi, S., & Hewes, S. (1994). Affective communication between mothers and preschoolers: Relations with social-emotional competence. *Merrill–Palmer Quarterly, 40,* 488–508.

Denham, S. A., Zahn-Waxler, C., Cummings, E. M., & Iannotti, R. J. (1991). Social competence in young children's peer relationships: Patterns of development and change. *Child Psychiatry and Human Development, 22,* 29–43.

Denham, S. A., & Zoller, D. (1990). *"When Mommy's angry, I feel sad": Preschoolers' understanding of emotion and its socialization.* Poster presented at the biennial Conference on Human Development, Richmond, VA.

Denham, S. A., & Zoller, D. (1991). "When my hamster died, I cried": Preschoolers' attributions of the causes of emotions. *Journal of Genetic Psychology, 152,* 371–373.

Denham, S. A., Zoller, D., & Couchoud, E. A. (1994). Socialization of preschoolers' understanding of emotion. *Developmental Psychology, 30,* 928–936.

Dissanayake, C., Sigman, M., & Kasari, C. (1996). Long-term stability of individual differences in the emotional responsiveness of children with autism. *Journal of Child Psychology and Psychiatry, 37,* 461–467.

Dix, T. (1991). The affective organization of parenting: Adaptive and maladaptive processes. *Psychological Bulletin, 110,* 3–25.

Dodge, K. A., & Frame, C. L. (1982). Social cognitive biases and deficits in aggressive boys. *Child Development, 53,* 620–635.

Donaldson, S. K., & Westerman, M. A. (1986). Development of children's understanding of ambivalence and causal theories of emotions. *Developmental Psychology, 22,* 655–662.

Dunn, J. (1988). *The beginnings of social understanding.* Cambridge, MA: Harvard University Press.

Dunn, J. (1995). Children as psychologists: The later correlates of individual differences in understanding of emotions and other minds. *Cognition and Emotion, 9,* 187–201.

Dunn, J., Bretherton, I., & Munn, P. (1987). Conversations about feeling states between mothers and their young children. *Developmental Psychology, 23,* 132–139.

Dunn, J., & Brown, J. R. (1994). Affect expression in the family: Children's understanding of emotions and their interactions with others. *Merrill–Palmer Quarterly, 40,* 120–137.

Dunn, J., Brown, J. R., & Beardsall, L. (1991). Family talk about feeling states and children's later understanding of others' emotions. *Developmental Psychology,* *27,* 448–455.

Dunn, J., Brown, J. R., & Maguire, M. (1995). The development of children's moral sensibility: Individual differences and emotion understanding. *Developmental Psychology, 31,* 649–659.

Dunn, J., Brown, J. R., Slomkowski, C., Tesla, C., & Youngblade, L. (1991). Young children's understanding of other people's feelings and beliefs: Individual differences and their antecedents. *Child Development, 62,* 1352–1366.

Dunn, J., & Hughes, C. (1998). Young children's understanding of emotions within close relationships. *Cognition and Emotion, 12,* 171–190.

Dunn, J., & Munn, P. (1985). Becoming a family member: Family conflict and the development of social understanding in the second year. *Child Development, 56,* 480–492.

During, S. M., & McMahon, R. J. (1991). Recognition of emotional facial expressions by abusive mothers and their children. *Journal of Clinical Child Psychology, 20,* 132–139.

Egeland, B., Kalkoske, M., Gottesman, N., & Erickson, M. F. (1990). Preschool behavior problems: Stability and factors accounting for change. *Journal of Child Psychology and Psychiatry, 31,* 891–909.

Eisenberg, N. (1986). *Altruism, emotion, cognition, and behavior.* Hillsdale, NJ: Erlbaum.

Eisenberg, N., Bernzweig, J., & Fabes, R. A. (1991). Coping and vicarious emotional responding. In T. M. Field, P. M. McCabe, & N. Schneiderman (Eds.), *Stress and coping in infancy and childhood* (pp. 101–117). Hillsdale, NJ: Erlbaum.

Eisenberg, N., & Fabes, R. A. (1992). Emotion, regulation, and the development of social competence. In M. S. Clark (Ed.), *Review of personality and social psychology: Vol. 14. Emotion and social behavior* (pp. 119–150). Newbury Park, CA: Sage.

Eisenberg, N., & Fabes, R. A. (1994). Mothers' reactions to children's negative emotions: Relations to children's temperament and anger behavior. *Merrill–Palmer Quarterly, 40,* 138–156.

Eisenberg, N., Fabes, R. A., Bernzweig, J., Karbon, M., Poulin, R., & Hanish, L. (1993). The relations of emotionality and regulation to preschoolers' social skills and sociometric status. *Child Development, 64,* 1418–1438.

Eisenberg, N., Fabes, R. A., Carlo, G., & Karbon, M. (1992). Emotional responsivity to others: Behavioral correlates and socialization antecedents. In N. Eisenberg & R. A. Fabes (Eds.), *New directions for child development: No. 55. Emotion and its regulation in early development* (pp. 57–73). San Francisco: Jossey-Bass.

Eisenberg, N., Fabes, R. A., Miller, P. A., Shell, R., Shea, C., & May-Plumlee, T. (1990). Preschoolers' vicarious emotional responding and their situational and dispositional prosocial behavior. *Merrill–Palmer Quarterly, 36,* 507–528.

Eisenberg, N., Fabes, R. A., Murphy, B., Karbon, M., Smith, M., & Maszk, P. (1996). The relations of children's dispositional empathy-related responding to their emotionality, regulation, and social functioning. *Developmental Psychology, 32,* 195–209.

Eisenberg, N., Fabes, R. A., Murphy, B., Maszk, P., Smith, M., & Karbon, M. (1995). The role of emotionality and regulation in children's social functioning: A longitudinal study. *Child Development, 66,* 1360–1384.

Eisenberg, N., Fabes, R. A., Nyman, M., Bernzweig, J., & Pinuelas, A. (1994). The relation of emotionality and regulation to preschoolers' anger-related reactions. *Child Development, 65,* 1352–1366.

Eisenberg, N., Fabes, R. A., Schaller, M., Carlo, G., & Miller, P. (1991). The relations of parental characteristics and practices to children's vicarious emotional responding. *Child Development, 62,* 1393–1408.

Eisenberg, N., McCreath, H., & Ahn, R. (1988). Vicarious emotional responsiveness and prosocial behavior: Their interrelations in young children. *Personality and Social Psychology Bulletin, 14,* 298–311.

Eisenberg, N., Pasternack, J. F., Cameron, E., & Tryon, K. (1984). The relations of quantity and mode of prosocial behavior to moral cognitions and social style. *Child Development, 55,* 1479–1485.

Eisenberg, N., Schaller, M., Fabes, R. A., Bustamante, D., Mathy, R., Shell, R., & Rhodes, K. (1988). Differentiation of personal distress and sympathy in children and adults. *Developmental Psychology, 24,* 766–775.

Ekman, P., & Friesen, W. V. (1975). *Unmasking the face.* Englewood Cliffs, NJ: Prentice-Hall.

El-Sheikh, M., Cummings, E. M., & Reiter, S. (1996). Preschoolers' responses to ongoing interadult conflict: The role of prior exposure to resolved versus unresolved arguments. *Journal of Abnormal Child Psychology, 24,* 665–679.

Emde, R. N., Bingham, R. D., & Harmon, R. J. (1993). Classification and the diagnostic process in infancy. In C. H. Zeanah (Ed.), *Handbook of infant mental health* (pp. 225–235). New York: Guilford Press.

Engel, S. (1995). *The stories children tell: Making sense of the narratives of childhood.* New York: W. H. Freeman.

Erickson, M. F., Egeland, B., & Pianta, R. (1989). The effects of maltreatment on the development of young children. In D. Cicchetti & V. Carlson (Eds.), *Child maltreatment: Theory and research on the courses and consequences of child abuse and neglect* (pp. 647–684). New York: Cambridge University Press.

Fabes, R. A., & Eisenberg, N. (1992). Young children's coping with interpersonal anger. *Child Development, 63,* 116–128.

Fabes, R. A., Eisenberg, N., & Bernzweig, J. (1990). *The Coping with Children's Negative Emotions Scale: Description and scoring.* Unpublished manuscript, Arizona State University.

Fabes, R. A., Eisenberg, N., Karbon, M., Bernzweig, J., Speer, A. L., & Carlo, G. (1994). Socialization of children's vicarious emotional responding and prosocial behavior: Relations with mothers' perceptions of children's emotional reactivity. *Developmental Psychology, 30,* 44–55.

Fabes, R. A., Eisenberg, N., McCormick, S. E., & Wilson, M. S. (1988). Preschoolers' attributions of the situational determinants of others' naturally occurring emotions. *Developmental Psychology, 24,* 376–385.

Fabes, R. A., Eisenberg, N., & Miller, P. A. (1990). Maternal correlates of children's vicarious emotional responsiveness. *Developmental Psychology, 26,* 639–648.

Fabes, R. A., Eisenberg, N., Nyman, M., & Michealieu, Q. (1991). Young children's appraisal of others' spontaneous emotional reactions. *Developmental Psychology, 27,* 858–866.

Farver, J. M., & Branstetter, W. H. (1994). Preschoolers' prosocial responses to their peers' distress. *Developmental Psychology, 30,* 334–341.

Felleman, E. S., Barden, R. C. Carlson, C. R., Rosenberg, L., & Masters, J. C. (1983). Children's and adults' recognition of spontaneous and posed emotional expressions in young children. *Developmental Psychology, 19,* 405–413.

Ferguson, T. (1996). *Self-report, narrative, and projective indicators of (mal)adaptive features of guilt and shame.* Paper presented at the biennial meeting of the International Society for Research in Emotions, Toronto.

Ferguson, T., Eyre, H. L., Stegge, H., Sorenson, C. B., & Everton, R. (1997). *The distinct roles of shame and guilt in childhood psychopathology.* Poster presented at the biennial meeting of the Society for Research in Child Development, Washington, DC.

Ferguson, T., & Stegge, H. (1995). Emotional states and traits in children: The case of guilt and shame. In J. P. Tangney & K. W. Fischer (Eds.), *Self-conscious emotions: The psychology of shame, guilt, embarrassment, and pride* (pp. 174–197). New York: Guilford Press.

Feshbach, N., & Cohen, S. (1988). Training affect comprehension in young children: An experimental evaluation. *Journal of Applied Developmental Psychology, 9,* 201–210.

Field, T. M., & Walden, T. A. (1982). Production and discrimination of facial expressions by preschool children. *Child Development, 53,* 1299–1311.

Fischer, K. W., Shaver, P. R., & Carnochan, P. (1989). A skill approach to emotional development: From basic- to superordinate-category emotions. In W. Damon (Ed.), *Child development today and tomorrow* (pp. 107–136). San Francisco: Jossey-Bass.

Fivush, R. (1989). Exploring sex differences in the emotional content of mother–child conversations about the past. *Sex Roles, 20,* 675–691.

Fogel, A., & Reimers, M. (1989). On the psychobiology of emotions and their development. *Monographs of the Society for Research in Child Development, 54*(1–2, Serial No. 219) 105–113.

Folkman, S. (1991). Coping across the life span: Theoretical issues. In E. M. Cummings, A. L. Greene, & K. H. Karraker (Eds), *Lifespan developmental psychology: Perspectives on stress and coping* (pp. 3–19). Hillsdale, NJ: Erlbaum.

Frankenburg, W. K., Camp, B. W., & Van Natta, P. A. (1971). Validity of the Denver Developmental Screening Test. *Child Development, 42,* 475–485.

Frankenburg, W. K., Dodds, J. B., Fandal, A. W., Kazuk, E., & Cohrs, M. (1975). *Denver Developmental Screening Test.* Denver, CO: Denver Developmental Materials.

Fuchs, D., & Thelen, M. H. (1988). Children's expected interpersonal consequences of communicating their affective state and reported likelihood of expression. *Child Development, 59,* 1314–1322.

Gardner, F. E. M. (1989). Inconsistent parenting: Is there evidence for a link with children's conduct problems? *Journal of Abnormal Child Psychology, 17*, 223–233.

Garner, P. W. (1995). Toddlers' emotion regulation behaviors: The role of social context and family expressiveness. *Journal of Genetic Psychology, 156*, 417–430.

Garner, P. W., Jones, D. C., Gaddy, G., & Rennie, K. (1997). Low income mothers' conversations about emotions and their children's emotional competence. *Social Development, 6*, 37–52.

Garner, P. W., Jones, D. C., & Miner, J. L. (1994). Social competence among low-income preschoolers: Emotion socialization practices and social cognitive correlates. *Child Development, 65*, 622–637.

Garner, P. W., Jones, D. C., & Palmer, D. J. (1994). Social cognitive correlates of preschool children's sibling caregiving behavior. *Developmental Psychology, 30*, 905–911.

Garner, P. W., & Power, T. G. (1996). Preschoolers' emotional control in the disappointment paradigm and its relation to temperament, emotion knowledge, and family expressiveness. *Child Development, 67*, 1406–1419.

Garner, P. W., Robertson, S., & Smith, G. (1997). Preschool children's emotional expressions with peers: The roles of gender and emotion socialization. *Sex Roles, 36*, 675–691.

George, C., & Main, M. (1979). Social interactions of young abused children: Approach, avoidance, and aggression. *Child Development, 50*, 306–318.

Gergen, K. J. (1985). The social constructionist movement in modern psychology. *American Psychologist, 40*, 266–275.

Gnepp, J. (1983). Children social sensitivity: Inferring emotions from conflicting cues. *Developmental Psychology, 19*, 805–814.

Gnepp, J. (1989a). Children's use of personal information to understand other people's feelings. In P. Harris & C. Saarni (Eds.), *Children's understanding of emotion* (pp. 151–177). Cambridge, England: Cambridge University Press.

Gnepp, J. (1989b). Personalized inferences of emotions and appraisals: Component processes and correlates. *Developmental Psychology, 25*, 277–288.

Gnepp, J., & Chilamkurti, C. (1988). Children's use of personality attributions to predict other people's emotional and behavioral reactions. *Child Development, 59*, 743–754.

Gnepp, J., & Gould, M. E. (1985). The development of personalized inferences: Understanding other people's emotional reactions in light of their prior experiences. *Child Development, 56*, 1455–1464.

Gnepp, J., & Hess, D. L. R. (1986). Children's understanding of verbal and facial display rules. *Developmental Psychology, 22*, 103–108.

Gnepp, J., Klayman, J., & Trabasso, T. (1982). A hierarchy of information sources for inferring emotional reactions. *Journal of Experimental Child Psychology, 33*, 111–123.

Gnepp, J., McKee, E., & Domanic, J. A. (1987). Children's use of situational information to infer emotion: Understanding emotionally equivocal situations. *Developmental Psychology, 23*, 114–123.

Goldman, J. A., Corsini, D. A., & de Urioste, R. (1980). Implications of positive and negative sociometric status for assessing social competence of young children. *Journal of Applied Developmental Psychology, 1,* 209–220.

Goleman, D. (1995). *Emotional intelligence.* New York: Bantam Books.

Gordis, F., Rosen, A. B., & Grand, S. (1989). *Young children's understanding of simultaneous conflicting emotions.* Poster presented at the biennial meeting of the Society for Research in Child Development, Kansas City, MO.

Gordon, S. L. (1989). The socialization of children's emotions: Emotional culture, competence, and exposure. In P. Harris & C. Saarni (Eds.), *Children's understanding of emotion* (pp. 319–349). Cambridge, England: Cambridge University Press.

Gotlieb, H., Lennox, C., Kronitz, Alan, M., Hart, J., & Read, E. (1993). *The Kindergarten intervention project: Facilitating the development of children's prosocial behaviors.* Paper presented at the biennial meeting of the Society for Research in Child Development, New Orleans, LA.

Gottman, J. M., & Katz, L. F. (1989). Effects of marital discord on young children's peer interaction and health. *Developmental Psychology, 25,* 373–381.

Gottman, J. M., Katz, L. F., & Hooven, C. (1996a). *Meta-emotion: How families communicate emotionally, links to child peer relations, and other developmental outcomes.* Mahwah, NJ: Erlbaum.

Gottman, J. M., Katz, L. F., & Hooven, C. (1996b). Parental meta-emotion philosophy and the emotional life of families: Theoretical model and preliminary data. *Journal of Family Psychology, 10,* 249–268.

Gould, M. E. (1984). *Children's recognition and resolution of ambiguity in making affective judgements.* Paper presented at the annual meeting of the Midwestern Psychological Association, Chicago.

Gove, F., & Keating, D. P. (1979). Empathic role-taking precursors. *Developmental Psychology, 15,* 594–600.

Gramzow, R., & Tangney, J. P. (1992). Proneness to shame and the narcissistic personality. *Personality and Social Psychology Bulletin, 18,* 369–376.

Greenberg, M. T., DeKlyen, M., & Speltz, M. L. (1989). *The relationship of insecure attachment to externalizing behavior problems in the preschool years.* Paper presented at the biennial meeting of the Society for Research in Child Development, Kansas City, MO.

Greenberg, M. T., Kusché, C. A., Cook E. T., & Quamma, J. P. (1995). Promoting emotional competence in school-aged children: The effects of the PATHS curriculum. *Development and Psychopathology, 7,* 117–136.

Greenspan, S. I. (1992). *Infancy and early childhood: The practice of clinical assessment and intervention with emotional and developmental challenges.* Madison, CT: International Universities Press.

Greenspan, S. (1994). Diagnostic classification of mental health and developmental disorders of infancy and early childhood. *Zero to Three, 14,* 34–41.

Greif, E. B., Alvarez, M., & Tone, M. (1984). *Parents' teaching of emotions to preschool children.* Paper presented at the annual meeting of the Eastern Psychological Association, Baltimore.

Grolnick, W. S, Bridges, L. J., & Connell, J. P. (1996). Emotion regulation in two-year-olds: Strategies and emotional expression in four contexts. *Child Development, 67,* 928–941.

Grolnick, W. S., McMenamy, J., Kurowski, C., & Bridges, L. J. (1997). *Mothers' strategies for regulating children's distress: Developmental changes and outcomes.* Paper presented at the biennial meeting of the Society for Research in Child Development, Washington, DC.

Gross, D. (1993). *Young children's understanding of misleading emotional displays.* Poster presented at the biennial meetings of the Society for Research in Child Development, New Orleans, LA.

Gross, D., & Harris, P. (1988). Understanding false beliefs about emotion. *International Journal of Behavioral Development, 11,* 475–488.

Grusec, J. E., & Goodnow, J. J. (1994). Impact of parental discipline methods on the child's internalization of values: A reconceptualization of current points of view. *Developmental Psychology, 30,* 4–19.

Hadwin, J., & Perner, J. (1991). Pleased and surprised: Children's cognitive theory of emotion. *British Journal of Developmental Psychology, 9,* 215–234.

Halberstadt, A. G. (1991). Socialization of expressiveness: Family influences in particular and a model in general. In R. S. Feldman & S. Rimé (Eds.), *Fundamentals of emotional expressiveness* (pp. 106–162). Cambridge, England: Cambridge University Press.

Halberstadt, A. G., & Fox, N. A. (1990). *Mothers' and their children's expressiveness and emotionality.* Poster presented at the biennial Conference on Human Development, Richmond, VA.

Halpern, L. F. (1997). *Preschoolers' coping with stressful events: Implications for psychological adjustment.* Poster presented at the biennial meeting of the Society for Research in Child Development, Washington, DC.

Harris, P. L. (1983). Children's understanding of the link between situation and emotion. *Journal of Experimental Child Psychology, 36,* 490–509.

Harris, P. L. (1989). *Children and emotion: The development of psychological understanding.* Oxford: Blackwell.

Harris, P. L. (1993). Understanding of emotions. In M. Lewis & J. Haviland (Eds.), *Handbook of emotions* (pp. 237–246). New York: Guilford Press.

Harris, P. L., Johnson, C. N., Hutton, D., Andrews, G. M., & Cooke, T. (1989). Young children's theory of mind and emotion. *Cognition and Emotion, 3,* 379–400.

Harter, S., & Buddin, B. J. (1987). Children's understanding of the simultaneity of two emotions: A five-stage developmental acquisition sequence. *Developmental Psychology, 23,* 388–399.

Harter, S., & Whitesell, N. R. (1989). Developmental changes in children's understanding of single, multiple, and blended emotion concepts. In P. Harris & C. Saarni (Eds.), *Children's understanding of emotion* (pp. 81–116). Cambridge, England: Cambridge University Press.

Henshaw, S. P., & Melnick, S. M. (1995). Peer relationships in boys with attention-deficit hyperactivity disorder with and without comorbid aggression. *Development and Psychopathology, 7,* 622–647.

Hertzig, M. E., Snow, M. E., & Sherman, M. (1989). Affect and cognition in autism. *Journal of the American Academy of Child and Adolescent Psychiatry, 28,* 195–199.

Hochschild, A. R. (1979). Emotion work, feeling rules, and social structure. *American Journal of Sociology, 85,* 551–575.

Hoffman, M. L. (1975). Altruistic behavior and the parent–child relationship. *Journal of Personality and Social Psychology, 31,* 937–943.

Hoffman, M. L. (1984). Interaction of affect and cognition in empathy. In C. E. Izard, J. Kagan, & R. B. Zajonc (Eds.), *Emotions, cognition, and behavior* (pp. 103–131). Cambridge, England: Cambridge University Press.

Hoffman, M. L., & Saltzstein, H. D. (1967). Parent discipline and the child's moral development. *Journal of Personality and Social Psychology, 5,* 45–57.

Hoffner, C., & Badzinski, D. M. (1989). Children's integration of facial and situations cues to emotion. *Child Development, 60,* 415–422.

Hooven, C., Katz, L., & Gottman, J. M. (1994). The family as a meta-emotion culture. *Cognition and Emotion, 9,* 229–264.

Howe, N. (1991). Sibling-directed internal state language, perspective-taking, and affective behavior. *Child Development, 62,* 1503–1512.

Howes, C., & Eldredge, R. (1985). Responses of abused, neglected, and non-maltreated children to the behaviors of their peers. *Journal of Applied Developmental Psychology, 6,* 261–270.

Howes, C., & Matheson, C. C. (1992). Contextual constraints on the concordance of mother–child and teacher–child relationships. In R. C. Pianta (Ed.), *New directions for child development: No. 57. Beyond the parent: The role of other adults in children's lives* (pp. 25–40). San Francisco: Jossey-Bass.

Hughes, M., & Kasari, C. (1995). *Caregiver child interactions and the expression of pride in children with Down syndrome.* Unpublished manuscript.

Hyson, M. C. (1994). *The emotional development of young children: Building an emotion-centered curriculum.* New York: Teachers College Press.

Hyson, M. C., & Lee, K.-M. (1996). Assessing early childhood teachers' beliefs about emotions: Content, contexts, and implications for practice. *Early Education and Development, 7,* 59–78.

Izard, C. E. (1991). *The psychology of emotions.* New York: Plenum Press.

Izard, C. E. (1993a). Four systems for emotion activation: Cognitive and noncognitive processes. *Psychological Review, 100,* 68–90.

Izard, C. E. (1993b). Organizational and motivational functions of discrete emotions. In M. Lewis & J. Haviland (Eds.), *Handbook of emotions* (pp. 631–642). New York: Guilford Press.

Izard, C. E., Dougherty, L., & Hembree, E. A. (1980). *System for identifying affect expressions by holistic judgment (AFFEX).* Newark: University of Delaware, Instructional Resources Center.

Jones, D. C., Abbey, B., & Cumberland, A. (in press). The development of display rule knowledge: Linkages with family expressiveness and social competence. *Child Development.*

Josephs, I. (1994). Display rule behavior and understanding in preschool children. *Journal of Nonverbal Behavior, 18,* 301–326.

Kasari, C., Hughes, M., & Freeman, S. (1994, June), *Emotion recognition in children with Down syndrome.* Paper presented at the biennial meeting of the International Society for the Study of Behavioural Development, Amsterdam.

Kasari, C., Mundy, P., & Sigman, M. (1991). *Empathy in toddlers with Down syndrome.* Paper presented at the biennial meeting of the Society for Research in Child Development, Seattle, WA.

Kasari, C., Mundy, P., Yirmiya, N., & Sigman, M. (1990). Affect and attention in children with Down syndrome. *American Journal on Mental Retardation, 95,* 55–67.

Kasari, C., & Sigman, M. (1996). Expression and understanding of emotion in atypical development: Autism and Down syndrome. In M. Lewis & M. E. Sullivan (Eds.), *Emotional development in atypical children* (pp. 109–130). Hillsdale, NJ: Erlbaum.

Kasari, C., Sigman, M., Baumgartner, P., & Stipek, D. (1993). Pride and mastery in children with autism. *Journal of Child Psychology and Psychiatry, 34,* 353–362.

Kenealy, P. (1989). Children's strategies for coping with depression. *Behaviour Research and Therapy, 27,* 27–34.

Kestenbaum, R., Farber, E. A., & Sroufe, L. A. (1989). Individual differences in empathy among preschoolers: Relation to attachment history. In N. Eisenberg & R. A. Fabes (Eds.), *New directions for child development: No. 44. Emotion and its regulation in early development* (pp. 51–64). San Francisco: Jossey-Bass.

Kestenbaum, R., & Gelman, S. (1995). Preschool children's identification and understanding of mixed emotions. *Cognitive Development, 10,* 443–458.

Kiselica, M. S., & Levin, G. R. (1987). *Young children's responses to a crying peer.* Paper presented at the biennial meeting of the Society for Research in Child Development, Baltimore.

Klimes-Dougan, B., & Kistner, J. (1990). Physically abused preschoolers' responses to peers' distress. *Developmental Psychology, 26,* 599–602.

Knitzer, J. (1993). Children's mental health policy: Challenging the future. *Journal of Emotional and Behavioral Disorders, 1,* 8–16.

Kochanska, G. (1987). *Socialization of young children's anger by well and depressed mothers.* Paper presented at the biennial meeting of the Society for Research in Child Development, Baltimore.

Kochanska, G., Casey, R. J., & Fukumoto, A. (1995). Toddlers' sensitivity to standard violations. *Child Development, 66,* 643–656.

Kopp, C. B. (1989). Regulation of distress and negative emotions: A developmental view. *Developmental Psychology, 25,* 343–354.

Kopp, C. B. (1994). *Baby steps: The "whys" of your child's behavior in the first two years.* New York: W. H. Freeman.

Kuebli, J., Butler, S., & Fivush, R. (1995). Mother–child talk about past emotions: Relations of maternal language and child gender over time. *Cognition and Emotion, 9,* 265–283.

Kuebli, J., & Fivush, R. (1992). Gender differences in parent–child conversations about past emotions. *Sex Roles, 27,* 683–698.

Kuebli, J., & Fivush, R. (1996). Making everyday events emotional: The construal of emotion in parent–child conversations about the past. In N. L. Stein, P. A. Ornstein, B. Tversky, & C. J. Brainerd (Eds.), *Memory for everyday and emotional events* (pp. 15–48). Mahwah, NJ: Erlbaum.

Kusché, C. A., & Greenberg, M. T. (1995a). *Promoting social and emotional development in deaf children: The PATHS project.* Seattle: University of Washington Press.

Kusché, C. A., & Greenberg, M. K. (1995b). *The PATHS curriculum.* Seattle, WA: Developmental Research and Programs.

LaFreniere, P. J., & Dumas, J. (1996). Social Competence and Behavior Evaluation in children aged three to six: The Short Form (SCBE-30). *Psychological Assessment, 8,* 369–377.

LaFreniere, P. J., Dumas, J. E., Capuano, F., & Dubeau, D. (1992). Development and validation of the Preschool Socioaffective Profile. *Psychological Assessment, 4,* 442–450.

LaFreniere, P. J., & Sroufe, L. A. (1985). Profiles of peer competence in the preschool: Interrelations between measures, influence of social ecology, and relation to attachment history. *Developmental Psychology, 21,* 46–69.

Lagattuta, K. H., Wellman, H. M., & Flavell, J. H. (1997). Preschoolers' understanding of the link between thinking and feeling: Cognitive cueing and emotional change. *Child Development, 68,* 1081–1104.

Lazarus, R. S. (1991). Cognition and motivation in emotion. *American Psychologist, 46,* 352–367.

LeDoux, J. (1993). Emotional networks in the brain. In M. Lewis & J. Haviland (Eds.), *Handbook of emotions* (pp. 109–118). New York: Guilford Press.

Lemerise, E. A., & Dodge, K. A. (1993). The development of anger and hostile interactions. In M. Lewis & J. Haviland (Eds.), *Handbook of emotions* (pp. 537–546). New York: Guilford Press.

Lemerise, E. A., & Gentil, J. (1992). Social competence: What is it and where does emotion fit in? In E. A. Lemerise & T. A. Walden (Chairs), *What can emotion variables contribute to our understanding of social competence?* Symposium presented at the biennial Conference on Human Development, Atlanta, GA

Lemerise, E., Scott, M. B., Diehl, D., & Bacher, B. (1996). *Understanding the emotions of victims and victimizers: Developmental, peer acceptance, and aggression level effects.* Manuscript submitted for publication.

Lemerise, E., Walden, T., & Smith, M. (1997). Contributions of emotion to preschool children's peer acceptance and friendship. In J. Hubbad (Chair), *The role of emotions in children's peer relationships.* Symposium conducted at the biennial meeting of the Society for Research in Child Development, Washington, DC.

Lennon, R., & Eisenberg, N. (1987). Emotional displays associated with preschoolers' prosocial behavior. *Child Development, 58,* 992–1000.

Lennon, R., Eisenberg, N., & Carroll, J. (1986). The relation between nonverbal indices of empathy and preschoolers' prosocial behavior. *Journal of Applied Developmental Psychology, 7,* 219–224.

Lewis, M. (1992). *Shame: The exposed self.* New York: Plenum Press.

Lewis, M. (1993a). Basic psychological processes in emotion. In M. Lewis & J. M. Haviland (Eds.), *Handbook of emotions* (pp. 223–236). New York: Guilford Press.

Lewis, M. (1993b). The development of deception. In M. Lewis & C. Saarni (Eds.), *Lying and deception in everyday life* (pp. 90–105). New York: Guilford Press.

Lewis, M., Alessandri, S. M., & Sullivan, M. (1992). Differences in shame and pride as a function of children's gender and task difficulty. *Child Development, 63,* 630–638.

Lewis, M., & Michalson, L. (1983). *Children's emotions and moods: Developmental theory and measurement.* New York: Plenum Press.

Lewis, M., Stanger, C., & Sullivan, M. (1989). Deception in three-year-olds. *Developmental Psychology, 25,* 439–443.

Lewis, M., Stanger, C., Sullivan, M., & Barone, P. (1991). Changes in embarrassment as a function of age, sex, and situation. *British Journal of Developmental Psychology, 9,* 485–492.

Lewis, M., Sullivan, M., Stanger, C., & Weiss, M. (1989). Self development and self-conscious emotions. *Child Development, 60,* 146–156.

Lewis, M., Sullivan, M., & Vasen, A. (1987). Making faces: Age and emotion differences in the posing of emotional expressions. *Developmental Psychology, 23,* 690–697.

Lieberman, A. (1993). *The emotional life of the toddler.* New York: Macmillan.

Lord, C., & Magill-Evans, J. (1995). Peer interactions of autistic children and adolescents. *Development and Psychopathology, 7,* 611–626.

Lynch, M., & Cicchetti, D. (1992). Maltreated children's reports of relatedness to their teachers. In R. C. Pianta (Ed.), *New directions for child development: No. 57. Beyond the parent: The role of other adults in children's lives* (pp. 81–108). San Francisco: Jossey-Bass.

Maccoby, E. (1983). Social-emotional development and response to stressors. In N. Garmezy & M. Rutter (Eds.), *Stress, coping, and development in children* (pp. 217–234). New York: McGraw-Hill.

Maccoby, E., & Martin, J. (1983). Socialization in the context of the family: Parent–child interaction. In P. H. Mussen (Series Ed.) & E. M. Hetherington (Vol. Ed.), *Handbook of child psychology: Vol. 4. Socialization, personality, and social development* (4th ed., pp. 1–101). New York: Wiley.

Main, M., & George, C. (1985). Responses of abused and disadvantaged toddlers to distress in agemates: A study in the day care setting. *Developmental Psychology, 21,* 407–412.

Malatesta, C. Z. (1981). Infant emotion and the vocal affect lexicon. *Motivation and Emotion, 5,* 1–23.

Malatesta, C. Z. (1990). The role of emotions in the development and organization of personality. In R. A. Thompson (Ed.), *Nebraska Symposium on Motivation: Vol. 36. Socioemotional development* (pp. 1–56). Lincoln: University of Nebraska Press.

Malatesta, C. Z., Culver, C., Tesman, J. R., & Shepard, B. (1989). The development of emotional expression during the first two years of life. *Monographs of the Society for Research in Child Development, 54*(1–2, Serial No. 219).

Malatesta, C. Z., & Haviland, J. M. (1982). Learning display rules: The socialization of emotion expression in infancy. *Child Development, 53,* 991–1003.

Malatesta-Magai, C., Leak, S., Tesman, J., Shepard, B., Culver, C., & Smaggia, B. (1994). Profiles of emotional development: Individual differences in facial and vocal expression of emotion during the second and third years of life. *International Journal of Behavioral Development, 17,* 239–269.

Marcus, R. F. (1980). Empathy and popularity. *Child Study Journal, 10*, 133–145.

Marcus, R. F. (1987). The role of affect in children's cooperation. *Child Study Journal, 17*, 153–168.

Mason, T., Mitchell-Copeland, J., & Denham, S. A. (1996). *Preschoolers' affective responses to adult sadness, anger, and pain.* Manuscript submitted for publication.

Matas, L., Arend, R. A., & Sroufe, L. A. (1978). Continuity of adaptation in the second year: The relationship between quality of attachment and later competence. *Child Development, 49*, 547–556.

McCoy, C. L., & Masters, J. C. (1985). The development of children's strategies for the social control of emotion. *Child Development, 56*, 1214–1222.

McGee, G. G., Feldman, R. S., & Chernin, L. (1991). A comparison of emotional facial display by children with autism and typical preschoolers. *Journal of Early Intervention, 15*, 237–245.

Miller, P. J., & Sperry, L. L. (1987). The socialization of anger and aggression. *Merrill–Palmer Quarterly, 33*, 1–31.

Miller, P. J., & Sperry, L. L. (1988). The socialization and acquisition of emotional meanings, with special reference to language: A reply to Saarni. *Merrill–Palmer Quarterly, 34*, 217–222.

Miller, S. M., & Green, M. L. (1985). Coping with stress and frustration: Origins, nature, and development. In M. Lewis & C. Saarni (Eds.), *The socialization of emotions* (pp. 263–314). New York: Plenum Press.

Morales, M., & Bridges, L. J. (1997). *Associations between parental attitude and the development of emotion regulation.* Poster presented at biennial meeting of the the Society for Research in Child Development, Washington, DC.

Moskowitz, C. (1997). *Self-evaluation.* Unpublished doctoral dissertation, George Mason University, Fairfax, VA.

Mundy, P., Kasari, C., & Sigman, M. (1992). Nonverbal communication, affective sharing, and intersubjectivity. *Infant Behavior and Development, 15*, 377–381.

Murgatroyd, S. J., & Robinson, E. J. (1993). Children's judgments of emotions following moral transgression. *International Journal of Behavioral Development, 16*, 93–111.

National Center for Clinical Infant Programs. (1993). *Classification of mental health and developmental disorders of infancy and early childhood.* Arlington, VA: Author.

Nunner-Winkler, G., & Sodian, B. (1988). Children's understanding of moral emotions. *Child Development, 59*, 1323–1338.

O'Neill, D. K., Astington, J. W., & Flavell, J. H. (1992). Young children's understanding of the role that sensory experiences play in knowledge acquisition. *Child Development, 63*, 474–490.

Parke, R. D., Cassidy, J., Burks, V. M., Carson, J. L., & Boyum, L. (1992). Familial contribution to peer competence among young children: The role of interactive and affective processes. In R. D. Parke & G. W. Ladd (Eds.), *Family–peer relationships: Modes of linkage* (pp. 107–134). Hillsdale, NJ: Erlbaum.

Parker, J. G., & Gottman, J. M. (1989). Social and emotional development in a relational context: Friendship interaction from early childhood to adolescence. In T. Berndt & G. Ladd (Eds.), *Peer relationships in child development* (pp. 95–131). New York: Wiley.

Parks, S. (1992). *Inside HELP–Hawaii Early Learning Profile administration and reference manual*. Palo Alto, CA: VORT.

Patterson, G. R. (1980). Mothers: The unacknowledged victims. *Monographs of the Society for Research in Child Development, 45*(5, Serial No. 186).

Patterson, G. R., Reid, J. B., & Dishion, T. J. (1992). *Antisocial boys*. Eugene, OR: Castalia.

Peng, M., Johnson, C. N., Pollock, J., Glasspool, R., & Harris, P. L. (1992). Training young children to acknowledge mixed emotions. *Cognition and Emotion, 6*, 387–401.

Philoppot, P., & Feldman, R. S. (1990). Age and social competence in pre-schoolers' decoding of facial expression. *British Journal of Social Psychology, 29*, 43–54.

Phillips, W., Baron-Cohen, S., & Rutter, M. (1995). To what extent can children with autism understand desire? *Development and Psychopathology, 7*, 151–169.

Phinney, J. S., Feshbach, N. D., & Farver, J. (1986). Preschool children's response to peer crying. *Early Childhood Research Quarterly, 1*, 207–219.

Reissland, J., & Harris, P. (1991). Children's use of display rules in pride-eliciting situations. *British Journal of Developmental Psychology, 9*, 431–435.

Richards, D. D., & Siegler, R. S. (1981). Very young children's acquisition of systematic problem-solving strategies. *Child Development, 52*, 1318–1321.

Ridgeway, D., & Kuczaj, S. (1985). Acquisition of emotion-descriptive language: Receptive and productive vocabulary norms for ages 18 months to 6 years. *Developmental Psychology, 21*, 901–908.

Ridley, C. A., & Bullock, D. D. (1984). Interpersonal problem-solving skills training with aggressive young children. *Journal of Applied Developmental Psychology, 5*, 213–223.

Ridley, C. A., Vaughn, S. R., & Wittman, S. K. (1982). Developing empathic skills: A model for preschool children. *Child Study Journal, 12*(2), 89–97.

Riese, M. L. (1990). Neonatal temperament in monozygotic and dizygotic twin pairs. *Child Development, 61*, 1230–1237.

Roberts, W. R., & Strayer, J. (1987). Parents' responses to the emotional distress of their children: Relations with children's competence. *Developmental Psychology, 23*, 415–422.

Robin, A. L., Schneider, M., & Dolnick, M. (1976). The Turtle Technique: An extended case study of self-control in the classroom. *Psychology in the Schools, 13*, 449–453.

Rogosch, F. A., Cicchetti, D., & Aber, J. L. (1995). The role of child maltreatment in early deviations in cognitive and affective processing abilities and later peer relationship problems. *Development and Psychopathology, 7*, 591–610.

Rubin, K. D., & Clark, M. L. (1983). Preschool teachers' ratings of behavioral problems: Observational, sociometric, and social-cognitive correlates. *Journal of Abnormal Child Psychology, 11*, 273–286.

Rubin, K. D., & Daniels-Byrness, T. (1983). Concurrent and predictive correlates of sociometric status in kindergarten and grade 1 children. *Merrill–Palmer Quarterly, 29*, 337–352.

Ruffman, T., & Keenan, T. R. (1996). The belief-based emotion of surprise: The case for a lag in understanding relative to false belief. *Developmental Psychology, 32,* 40–49.

Russell, J. A. (1989). Culture, scripts, and children's understanding of emotion. In P. P. Harris & C. Saarni (Eds.), *Children's understanding of emotion* (pp. 293–318). Cambridge, England: Cambridge University Press.

Russell, J. A. (1990). The preschooler's understanding of the causes and consequences of emotion. *Child Development, 61,* 1872–1881.

Russell, J. A. (1994). Is there universal recognition of emotion from facial expression?: A review of the cross cultural studies. *Psychological Bulletin, 115,* 102–141.

Russell, J. A., & Paris, F. A. (1994). Do children acquire concepts of complex emotions abruptly? *International Journal of Behavioral Development, 17,* 349–365.

Saarni, C. (1987). Cultural rules of emotional experience: A commentary on Miller and Sperry's study. *Merrill–Palmer Quarterly, 33,* 535–540.

Saarni, C. (1990). Emotional competence. In R. A. Thompson (Ed.), *Nebraska Symposium on Motivation: Vol. 36. Socioemotional development* (pp. 115–161). Lincoln: University of Nebraska Press.

Saarni, C., & von Salisch, M. (1993). The socialization of emotional dissemblance. In M. Lewis & C. Saarni (Eds.), *Lying and deception in everyday life* (pp. 106–125). New York: Guilford Press.

Sachs-Alter, E. (1989). *The contextual use of facial expressions by maltreating and nonmaltreating mothers.* Unpublished master's thesis, DePaul University, Chicago.

Sachs-Alter, E. (1993). *Maltreated and nonmaltreated children's use of cues in understanding the emotions of others.* Unpublished doctoral dissertation, DePaul University, Chicago.

Sawyer, K. S. (1996). *Sibling contributions to young children's emotional competence.* Unpublished doctoral dissertation, George Mason University, Fairfax, VA.

Schneider, M., & Robin, A. L. (1978). *Manual for the Turtle Technique.* Unpublished manual, Department of Psychology, State University of New York at Stony Brook.

Shatz, M. (1994). *A toddler's life: Becoming a person.* New York: Oxford University Press.

Shields, A. M., Cicchetti, D., & Ryan, R. M. (1994). The development of emotional and behavioral self-regulation and social competence among maltreated school age children. *Development and Psychopathology, 6,* 57–75.

Shure, M. B. (1990). *ICPS problem solving techniques for preschool age children for use by teachers* (2nd ed.). Philadelphia: Hahnemann University.

Shure, M. B., & Spivack, G. (1982). Interpersonal problem-solving in young children: A cognitive approach to prevention. *American Journal of Community Psychology, 10,* 341–356.

Siegler, R. S., & Jenkins, E. (1989). *How children discover new strategies.* Hillsdale, NJ: Erlbaum.

Sigman, M. D., Kasari, C., Kwon, J. H., & Yirmiya, N. (1992). Responses to the negative emotions of others by autistic, mentally retarded, and normal children. *Child Development, 63,* 796–807.

Smiley, P., & Huttenlocher, J. (1989). Young children's acquisitions of emotion concepts. In P. Harris & C. Saarni (Eds.), *Children's understanding of emotion* (pp. 27–79). Cambridge, England: Cambridge University Press.

Smith, M., & Walden, T. (in press). Developmental trends in emotion understanding among African-American preschool children. *Journal of Applied Developmental Psychology.*

Snow, M. E., Hertzig, M. E., & Shapiro, T. (1987). Expression of emotion in young autistic children. *Journal of the American Academy of Child and Adolescent Psychiatry, 26,* 836–838.

Sroufe, L. A., & Fleeson, J. (1986). Attachment and the construction of relationships. In W. Hartup & Z. Rubin (Eds.), *Relationships and development* (pp. 51–72). Hillsdale, NJ: Erlbaum.

Sroufe, L. A., Schork, E., Motti, F., Lawroski, N., & LaFreniere, P. (1984). The role of affect in social competence. In C. E. Izard, J. Kagan, & R. B. Zajonc (Eds.), *Emotions, cognition, and behavior* (pp. 289–319). Cambridge, England: Cambridge University Press.

Stansbury, K., & Sigman, M. (1995). *Development of behavioral expressions of emotion regulation in normally developing and at-risk preschool-age children.* Manuscript submitted for publication.

Stein, N., & Jewett, J. L. (1986). A conceptual analysis of the meaning of negative emotions: Implications for a theory of development. In C. E. Izard & P. Read (Eds.), *Measurement of emotions in children* (Vol. 2, pp. 238–268). New York: Cambridge University Press.

Stein, N., & Levine, L. (1989). The causal organization of emotional knowledge: A developmental study. *Cognition and Emotion, 3,* 343–378.

Stein, N., & Levine, L. (1990). Making sense out of emotion: The representation and use of goal-structured knowledge. In N. Stein, T. Leventhal, & T. Trabasso (Eds.), *Psychological and biological approaches to emotion* (pp. 45–74). Hillsdale, NJ: Erlbaum.

Stein, N., & Trabasso, T. (1989). Children's understanding of changing emotional states. In P. Harris & C. Saarni (Eds.), *Children's understanding of emotion* (pp. 50–80). Cambridge, England: Cambridge University Press.

Stein, N., Trabasso, T., & Liwag, M. (1993). The representation and organization of emotional experience: Unfolding the emotion episode. In M. Lewis & J. Haviland (Eds.), *Handbook of emotions* (pp. 279–300). New York: Guilford Press.

Stifter, C., & Fox, N. (1987). Preschoolers' ability to identify and label emotions. *Journal of Nonverbal Behavior, 10,* 255–266.

Stipek, D., Recchia, S., & McClintic, S. (1992). Self-evaluation in young children. *Monographs of the Society for Research in Child Development, 57*(1, Serial No. 226), 1–84.

Straker, G., & Jacobson, R. S. (1981). Aggression, emotional maladjustment, and empathy in the abused child. *Developmental Psychology, 17,* 762–765.

Strayer, J. (1980). A naturalistic study of empathic behaviors and their relation to affective states and perspective-taking skills in preschool children. *Child Development, 51,* 815-822.

Strayer, J. (1986). Children's attributions regarding the situational determinants of emotion in self and others. *Developmental Psychology, 22,* 649-654.

Strayer, J. (1993). Children's concordant emotions and cognitions in response to observed emotions. *Child Development, 64,* 188-210.

Strayer, J., & Schroeder, M. (1989). Children's helping strategies: Influences of emotion, empathy, and age. In N. Eisenberg (Ed.), *New directions for child development: No. 44. Empathy and related emotional responses* (pp. 85-105). San Francisco: Jossey-Bass.

Tangney, J. P. (1990). Assessing individual differences in proneness to shame and guilt: Development of the Self-Conscious Affect and Attribution Inventory. *Journal of Personality and Social Psychology, 59,* 102-111.

Tangney, J. P. (1991). Moral affect: The good, the bad, and the ugly. *Journal of Personality and Social Psychology, 61,* 598-607.

Tangney, J. P. (1992). Situational determinants of shame and guilt in young adulthood. *Personality and Social Psychology Bulletin, 18,* 199-206.

Tangney, J. P. (1995a). Shame and guilt in interpersonal relationships. In J. P. Tangney & K. W. Fischer (Eds.), *Self-conscious emotions: The psychology of shame, guilt, embarrassment, and pride.* New York: Guilford Press.

Tangney, J. P. (1995b). The mixed legacy of the super-ego: Adaptive and maladaptive aspects of shame and guilt. In J. M. Masling & R. R. Bornstein (Eds.), *Empirical studies of psychoanalytic theories* (Vol. 5, pp. 1-28). Washington, DC: American Psychological Association.

Tangney, J. P. (1996). *Assessing shame-proneness and guilt-proneness from middle childhood through adulthood.* Paper presented at the biennial meeting of the International Society for Research in Emotions, Toronto.

Tangney, J. P. (1998). How does guilt differ from shame? In J. A. Bybee (Ed.), *Guilt and children* (pp. 1-17). New York: Academic Press.

Tangney, J. P., Burggraf, S. A., & Wagner, P. E. (1995). Shame-proneness, guilt-proneness, and psychological symptoms. In J. P. Tangney & K. W. Fischer (Eds.), *Self-conscious emotions: The psychology of shame, guilt, embarrassment, and pride* (pp. 347-367). New York: Guilford Press.

Tangney, J. P., Flicker, L., Barlow, D. H., & Miller, R. S. (1996). Are shame, guilt, and embarrassment distinct emotions? *Journal of Personality and Social Psychology, 70,* 1256-1269.

Tangney, J. P., Wagner, P. E., Barlow, D. H., Marschall, D. E., Sanftner, J., Mohr, T., & Gramzow, R. (1996). The relation of shame and guilt to constructive vs. destructive responses to anger across the lifespan. *Journal of Personality and Social Psychology, 70,* 797-809.

Tangney, J. P., Wagner, P. E., Fletcher, C., & Gramzow, R. (1991). Intergenerational continuities and discontinuities in proneness to shame and proneness to guilt. In J. P. Tangney (Chair), *Socialization of emotion in the family.* Symposium conducted at the biennial meeting of the Society for Research in Child Development, Seattle, WA.

Tesman, J. R., Shepard, B., & VanValkenburgh, L. (1993). *Expressions of shame in five-year-old children*. Paper presented at the biennial meeting of the Society for Research in Child Development, New Orleans, LA.

Thompson, R. A. (1990). Emotion and self regulation. In R. A. Thompson (Ed.), *Nebraska Symposium on Motivation: Vol. 36. Socioemotional development* (pp. 367–468). Lincoln: University of Nebraska Press.

Thompson, R. A. (1993). Socioemotional development: Enduring issues and new challenges. *Developmental Review, 13,* 372–402.

Thompson, R. A. (1994). Emotion regulation: A theme in search of definition. In N. A. Fox (Ed.), The development of emotion regulation: Biological and behavioral considerations. *Monographs of the Society for Research in Child Development, 59*(2–3, Serial No. 240), 25–52.

Thompson, R. A., & Calkins, S. (1996). The double-edged sword: Emotional regulation for children at risk. *Development and Psychopathology, 8,* 163–182.

Tomkins, S. (1962). *Affect, imagery, and consciousness: Vol. 1. The positive affects.* New York: Springer.

Tomkins, S. (1963). *Affect, imagery, and consciousness: Vol. 2. The negative affects.* New York: Springer.

Tomkins, S. (1991). *Affect, imagery, and consciousness: Vol. 3. The negative affects: Anger and fear.* New York: Springer.

Toth, S. L., Manly, J., & Cicchetti, D. (1992). Child maltreatment and vulnerability to depression. *Development and Psychopathology, 4,* 97–112.

Tronick, E. (1989). Emotions and emotional communication in infants. *American Psychologist, 44,* 112–119.

van IJzendoorn, M. H., Sagi, A., & Lambermon, M. W. E. (1992). The multiple caretaker paradox: Data from Holland and Israel. In R. C. Pianta (Ed.), *New directions for child development: No. 57. Beyond the parent: The role of other adults in children's lives* (pp. 5–24). San Francisco: Jossey-Bass.

Vaughn, B. E., Contreras, J., & Seifer, R. (1993). Short-term longitudinal study of maternal ratings of temperament in samples of children with Down syndrome and children who are developing normally. *American Journal of Mental Retardation, 98,* 607–618.

Walden, T. A., & Field, T. (1990). Preschool children's social competence and production and discrimination of affective expressions. *British Journal of Developmental Psychology, 8,* 65–76.

Walden, T. A., Lemerise, E. A., & Gentil, J. (1992). *Emotional competence and peer acceptance among preschool children.* In E. A. Lemerise & T. A. Walden (Chairs), *What can emotion variables contribute to our understanding of social competence?* Symposium conducted at the biennial Conference on Human Development, Atlanta, GA.

Waters, E., & Sroufe, L. A. (1983). Social competence as a developmental construct. *Developmental Review, 3,* 79–97.

Waters, E., Wippman, J., & Sroufe, L. A. (1979). Two studies in construct validation: Attachment, positive affect, and competence in the peer group. *Child Development, 50,* 821–829.

Weinberger, N., & Bushnell, E. W. (1994). Young children's knowledge about their senses: Perceptions and misconceptions. *Child Study Journal, 24,* 209–235.

Wellman, H. M. (1990). *The child's theory of mind.* Cambridge, MA: MIT Press.

Wellman, H. M., & Banerjee, M. (1991). Mind and emotion: Children's understanding of the emotional consequences of beliefs and desires. *British Journal of Developmental Psychology, 9,* 191–214.

Wellman, H. M., & Woolley, J. D. (1990). From simple desires to ordinary beliefs: The early development of everyday psychology. *Cognition, 35,* 245–275.

Werner, E. E. (1989). High-risk children in young adulthood: A longitudinal study from birth to 32 years. *American Journal of Orthopsychiatry, 59,* 72–81.

Whissell, C. K., & Nicholson, H. (1991). Children's freely produced synonyms for seven key emotions. *Perceptual and Motor Skills, 72,* 1107–1111.

Whitesell, N. R. (1989). *A prototype approach to children's understanding of basic emotions.* Paper presented at the biennial meeting of the Society for Research in Child Development, Kansas City, MO.

Widlansky, H. (1994). *Children's gaze and mother's intonation: Possible mediators of children's expression recognition learning.* Unpublished master's thesis, DePaul University, Chicago.

Wiggers, M., & Van Lieshout, C. F. (1985). Development of recognition of emotions: Children's reliance on situational and facial expressive cues. *Developmental Psychology, 21,* 338–349.

Wilson, B. J., & Cantor, J. (1985). Developmental differences in empathy with a television protagonist's fear. *Journal of Experimental Psychology, 39,* 284–299.

Wintre, M., Polivy, J., & Murray, M. A. (1990). Self-predictions of emotional response patterns: Age, sex, and situational determinants. *Child Development, 61,* 1124–1133.

Wintre, M., & Vallance, D. D. (1994). A developmental sequence in the comprehension of emotions: Multiple emotions, intensity and valence. *Developmental Psychology, 30,* 509–514.

Yirmiya, N., Kasari, C., Sigman, M., & Mundy, P. (1989). Facial expression of affect in autistic, mentally retarded, and normal children. *Journal of Child Psychology and Psychiatry, 30,* 725–795.

Youngblade, L. M., & Dunn, J. (1995). Individual differences in young children's pretend play with mother and sibling: Links to relationships and understanding of other people's feelings and beliefs. *Child Development, 66,* 1472–1492.

Yuill, N. (1984). Young children's coordination of motive and outcome in judgements of satisfaction and morality. *British Journal of Developmental Psychology, 2,* 73–81.

Zahn-Waxler, C., Iannotti, R. J., Cummings, E. M., & Denham, S. A. (1990). Antecedents of problem behaviors in children of depressed mothers. *Development and Psychopathology, 3,* 271–292.

Zahn-Waxler, C., & Kochanska, G. (1990). The origins of guilt. In R. A. Thompson (Ed.), *Nebraska Symposium on Motivation: Vol. 36. Socioemotional development* (pp. 183–258). Lincoln: University of Nebraska Press.

Zahn-Waxler, C., Kochanska, G., Krupnick, J., & McKnew, D. (1990). Patterns of guilt in children of depressed and well mothers. *Developmental Psychology,* *26,* 51–59.

Zahn-Waxler, C., Mayfield, A., Radke-Yarrow, M., McKnew, D., Cytryn, L., & Davenport, Y. (1988). A follow-up investigation of offspring of bipolar parents. *American Journal of Psychiatry, 145,* 506–509.

Zahn-Waxler, C., McKnew, D., Cummings, E. M., Davenport, Y., & Radke-Yarrow, M. (1984). Problem behaviors and peer interactions of young children with a manic–depressive parent. *American Journal of Psychiatry, 141,* 236–240.

Zahn-Waxler, C., & Radke-Yarrow, M. (1982). The development of altruism: Alternative research strategies. In N. Eisenberg (Ed.), *The development of prosocial behavior* (pp. 109–137). New York: Academic Press.

Zahn-Waxler, C., & Radke-Yarrow, M. (1990). The origins of empathic concern. *Motivation and Emotion, 14,* 107–130.

Zahn-Waxler, C., Radke-Yarrow, M., & King, R. A. (1979). Child rearing and children's prosocial initiations toward victims of distress. *Child Development, 50,* 319–330.

Zahn-Waxler, C., Ridgeway, D., Denham, S. A., Usher, B., & Cole, P. (1993). Research strategies for assessing mothers' interpretations of infants' emotions. In R. Emde, J. Osofsky, & P. Butterfield (Eds.), *The IFEEL pictures: A new instrument for interpreting emotions* (pp. 217–236). Madison, CT: International Universities Press.

Zahn-Waxler, C., Robinson, J., & Emde, R. (1992). Development of empathy in twins. *Developmental Psychology, 28,* 1038–1047.

Zeaman, J., & Garber, J. (1996). Display rules for anger, sadness, and pain: It depends on who is watching. *Child Development, 67,* 957–973.

# Index

253